Orofacial Pain

Nalini Vadivelu • Amarender Vadivelu
Alan David Kaye
Editors

Orofacial Pain

A Clinician's Guide

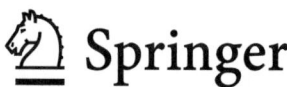

Editors
Nalini Vadivelu
Department of Anesthesiology
Yale University School of Medicine
   and Yale-New Haven Hospital
New Haven, CT, USA

Amarender Vadivelu
Department of Periodontology
Annoor Dental College
Kerala, India

Alan David Kaye
Departments of Anesthesiology
   and Pharmacology
LSU Health Sciences Center
New Orleans, LA, USA

LSU Interim Hospital
   and Ochsner Kenner Hospital
New Orleans, LA, USA

ISBN 978-3-319-01874-4   ISBN 978-3-319-01875-1 (eBook)
DOI 10.1007/978-3-319-01875-1
Springer Cham Heidelberg New York Dordrecht London

Library of Congress Control Number: 2013956820

© Springer International Publishing Switzerland 2014
This work is subject to copyright. All rights are reserved by the Publisher, whether the whole or part of the material is concerned, specifically the rights of translation, reprinting, reuse of illustrations, recitation, broadcasting, reproduction on microfilms or in any other physical way, and transmission or information storage and retrieval, electronic adaptation, computer software, or by similar or dissimilar methodology now known or hereafter developed. Exempted from this legal reservation are brief excerpts in connection with reviews or scholarly analysis or material supplied specifically for the purpose of being entered and executed on a computer system, for exclusive use by the purchaser of the work. Duplication of this publication or parts thereof is permitted only under the provisions of the Copyright Law of the Publisher's location, in its current version, and permission for use must always be obtained from Springer. Permissions for use may be obtained through RightsLink at the Copyright Clearance Center. Violations are liable to prosecution under the respective Copyright Law.
The use of general descriptive names, registered names, trademarks, service marks, etc. in this publication does not imply, even in the absence of a specific statement, that such names are exempt from the relevant protective laws and regulations and therefore free for general use.
While the advice and information in this book are believed to be true and accurate at the date of publication, neither the authors nor the editors nor the publisher can accept any legal responsibility for any errors or omissions that may be made. The publisher makes no warranty, express or implied, with respect to the material contained herein.

Printed on acid-free paper

Springer is part of Springer Science+Business Media (www.springer.com)

Foreword

Orofacial pain represents a problem that is common, unique, diverse in many ways, and challenging. Orofacial pain is *common* because it affects many millions of people worldwide. In the United States alone, more than 39 million adults, or 22 % of the adult population, report orofacial pain, and the magnitude is similar in several other countries where large population-based surveys have been carried out, including the United Kingdom and Germany. It is a problem not only of the developed but also of the developing countries, and it mandates the attention of scientists, clinicians, and public health policy makers because of its magnitude and costs in terms of healthcare, impaired productivity, and poor quality of life.

Orofacial pain is *unique* because the orofacial pain system, particularly the trigeminal pain system, has several distinctive features that distinguish it from the spinal pain system. These include electrophysiological, anatomical, biochemical, and pharmacological properties of trigeminal afferents innervating distinct target tissues. In the trigeminal system, for example, the proportion of myelinated to unmyelinated fibers and the properties of some of these fibers are different from those in spinal nerves. Further, there are sites in the orofacial region (e.g., tooth pulp, cornea) that are predominantly or exclusively innervated by nociceptive afferents. Even in the higher levels of the somatosensory system, there is bilateral and disproportionately large representation of the orofacial region.

Orofacial pain is *diverse* in many ways. It is derived from a diverse range of target tissues, such as the meninges, cornea, tooth pulp, oral/nasal mucosa, and the temporomandibular joint. Some of the uniqueness of the orofacial pain system derives from the distinctive characteristics of these target tissues. Thus, orofacial pain may arise from a wide variety of specific sites such as tooth and surrounding structures, temporomandibular joint, muscle, mucosa, sinus, bone, and salivary glands, or it may be referred from adjoining sites such as eyes, ear, intracranium, or even the heart. The etiology of orofacial pain may range from inflammatory to neuropathic to functional or idiopathic. Orofacial pain syndromes can be as diverse as their sites of origin, and more than twenty syndromes have been localized to the orofacial region including pulpitis, temporomandibular disorder, trigeminal neuralgia, and cluster headache just to name a few. Finally, the treatment approaches to various orofacial syndromes are diverse too, ranging from pharmacological, surgical, hypnotic, and cognitive-behavioral therapies.

It is not surprising, then, that orofacial pain presents an important *challenge* to scientists and clinicians alike. There have been significant strides in the recent past in our understanding, classification, and management of orofacial pain, but many questions remain. It is important to bring together the current state of the art and science in this area. *Orofacial Pain: A Clinician's Manual* essentially serves this very purpose. Many components of the book address etiology, epidemiology, and diagnosis to assist in guiding the clinician; then the book formally develops approaches to classification and measurement of orofacial pain and pain syndromes; and it concludes with treatment, management, and therapy modalities towards the multitude of aspects related to oral and facial pain. The editors have produced a text inclusive of solid reviews of basic and common oral health issues and facial pain disease processes as well as a source and reference for addressing more complex and future concerns. The book contains a broad table of contents inclusive of addressing fundamentals (anatomy, physiology, and pharmacology), proper assessment and classification of orofacial pain, along with both pharmacology and non-pharmacologic treatment approaches. The authors of the book, experts in their respective areas, address common clinical situations and also cover topics of interest such as epidemiology, pain management of patients with special needs, along with chapters addressing cognitive and behavioral complexities associated with orofacial pain and pain syndromes. This book should prove to be an essential tool in the armamentarium of those involved in the care of people suffering from orofacial pain syndromes in the developing and developed countries alike.

Chandigarh, India   Sukanya Mitra, M.D., M.A.M.S.

Preface

Orofacial pain can immensely affect the functionality of a human being since respirations, eating, chewing, swallowing, and speaking are vital functions all of which involve the orofacial area. Understanding orofacial pain and finding solutions to the treatment of this condition is a challenge. We have created an evidence based book with in-depth review of common clinical presentations, describing the appropriate history taking methods, as well as the detailed examinations and appropriate tests to help with diagnosis followed by medical and interventional managements to treat orofacial pain effectively. Multimodal approach is emphasized in every chapter.

This book has been written by several experts treating orofacial pain and covers a wide range of topics from acute to chronic orofacial pain. Topics include the classification and epidemiology of orofacial pain, nociceptive mediators, neurobiology of orofacial pain headache, oral ulcers, facial pain, headaches, neuropathic orofacial pain conditions, analgesics and adjuvant behavioral therapy, and interventional treatments.

This book is aimed toward health care professionals in all specialties as a valuable reference manual for the treatment of orofacial pain. We thank all our contributors for their excellent work, our colleagues and our families for their support. We would like to thank Nirmal Kumar Vadivelu, Gopal Kodumudi, Vijay Kodumudi and Rashmi Vadivelu for their assistance in the preparation of this manuscript. We would also like to acknowledge Ms. Asma Ahmed of Bentham Science publications and Dr. Rahul K. Arora, Dean, Oman Dental College, Muscat and Dr. Mohamed Al Ismaily, Chairman, Oman Dental College, Muscat for their encouragement and help.

New Haven, CT, USA	Nalini Vadivelu, M.D.
Muvattupuzha, Kerala, India	Amarender Vadivelu, B.D.S., M.D.S.
New Orleans, LA, USA	Alan David Kaye, M.D., Ph.D.

Contents

1 **The Neurobiology of Orofacial Pain**.. 1
   Nalini Vadivelu, Yili Huang, Peter Mancini, Shaun Gruenbaum,
   Amarender Vadivelu, and Susan Dabu-Bondoc

2 **Oral Health-Related Quality of Life and Facial Pain**...................... 9
   Amarender Vadivelu

3 **Classification and Epidemiology of Orofacial Pain** 15
   Suhas Setty and Jamil David

4 **Nociceptive Chemical Mediators in Oral Inflammation** 25
   Nalini Vadivelu, Anusha Manje Gowda, Stephen Thorp,
   Alice Kai, Amarender Vadivelu, and Susan Dabu-Bondoc

5 **Dental Sleep Medicine and the Use of Oral Devices** 35
   Ghabi A. Kaspo

6 **Local Anesthesia in the Orofacial Region** 65
   Thomas M. Halaszynski

7 **Analgesics and Adjuvants for the Management
   of Orofacial Pain Across Age Groups**.. 81
   Ian Laughlin and Anita H. Hickey

8 **Cognitive Behavioral Therapy in Pain Management** 89
   Thomas M. Halaszynski

9 **Management of Oral Ulcers and Burning Mouth Syndrome** 103
   Thomas M. Halaszynski

10 **Hypnosis and Biofeedback for Orofacial Pain Management**............. 115
   Janet Crain

11 **Headaches, Migraine, and Cluster Headache** 133
   Ghabi A. Kaspo

12	**Management of Orofacial Neuropathic Pain**..	143
	Subha Giri	
13	**Preemptive Analgesia and Multimodal Pain Management for Temporomandibular Total Joint Replacement Surgery**................	151
	Daniel B. Spagnoli and Alan David Kaye	
14	**Masticatory Myofascial Pain**	161
	Subha Giri	

Index... 173

Contributors

Janet Crain, D.M.D. The Center for Headaches, Facial Pain, and Sleep Apnea, South Amboy, NJ, USA

Susan Dabu-Bondoc, M.D. Department of Anesthesiology, Yale University School of Medicine, New Haven, CT, USA

Haven Hospital, New Haven, CT, USA

Jamil David, B.D.S., M.Sc., Ph.D. Department of Health Services Research, University of Liverpool, Liverpool, UK

Subha Giri, B.D.S., M.S. Minnesota Head and Neck Pain Clinic, Twin Cities, MN, USA

Anusha Manje Gowda, M.B.B.S. Bangalore Medical college and research institute, Bangalore, Karnataka, India

Shaun Gruenbaum, M.D. Department of Anesthesiology, Yale University School of Medicine, New Haven, CT, USA

Thomas M. Halaszynski, D.M.D., M.D., M.B.A. Department of Anesthesiology, Yale University School of Medicine and Yale-New Haven Hospital, New Haven, CT, USA

Anita H. Hickey, M.D. Naval Medical Center, San Diego, CA, USA

Yili Huang, D.O. Department of Anesthesiology, Yale University School of Medicine, New Haven, CT, USA

Alice Kai, B.A. Neuroplasticity Unit, National Institutes of Health, Bethesda, MD, USA

Ghabi A. Kaspo, D.D.S., D.Orth. Clinical instructor of the St. Joseph Hospital-Oakland Dental Residency Program, Staff at St. Joseph Mercy Hospital of Pontiac and Wayne State University, Troy, MI, USA

Wayne State University - Detroit Medical Centers, MI, USA

Alan David Kaye, M.D., Ph.D. Department of Anesthesiology, Louisiana State University School of Medicine, New Orleans, LA, USA

Department of Pharmacology, Louisiana State University School of Medicine, New Orleans, LA, USA

Ian Laughlin, M.D. Naval Medical Center, San Diego, CA, USA

Peter Mancini, M.D. Department of Anesthesiology, Yale University School of Medicine, New Haven, CT, USA

Daniel B. Spagnoli, D.D.S., M.S., Ph.D. Department of Oral and Maxillofacial Surgery, School of Dentistry, Louisiana State University Health Science Center, New Orleans, LA, USA

Suhas Setty, B.D.S., M.D.S. Department of Oral Medicine and Radiology, Sri Siddhartha Dental College, Tumkur, India

Stephen Thorp, M.D. Department of Anesthesiology, Yale University School of Medicine and Yale-New Haven Hospital, New Haven, CT, USA

Nalini Vadivelu, M.D. Department of Anesthesiology, Yale University School of Medicine and Yale-New Haven Hospital, New Haven, CT, USA

Amarender Vadivelu, B.D.S., M.D.S. Annoor Dental College and Hospital, Muvattupuzha, Kerala, India

Chapter 1
The Neurobiology of Orofacial Pain

Nalini Vadivelu, Yili Huang, Peter Mancini, Shaun Gruenbaum, Amarender Vadivelu, and Susan Dabu-Bondoc

Introduction

Pain is a health issue that affects many Americans. It is estimated that $6 billion is spent annually in the treatment of pain in the USA [1]. Pain disorders cause severe psychological, emotional, and social stresses and may interfere with activities of daily living and sleep, thereby perpetuating a vicious cycle of pain and social dysfunction.

The orofacial area holds special significance in daily actions such as eating, drinking, speech, and sexual behavior, and pain in that region is especially debilitating. The area is also richly innervated, and the influx of such sensations may be the reason why so many people find going to the dentist unpleasant [2]. There have been numerous recent advances in the understanding of the unique pathophysiology of orofacial pain, and this chapter details both neurologic pathways in which the pain is generated as well as the biochemical modalities by which the pain is modulated.

N. Vadivelu, M.D. (✉)
Department of Anesthesiology, Yale University School of Medicine and Yale-New Haven Hospital, 333 Cedar Street, 208051, New Haven, CT 06520-8051, USA
e-mail: Nalinivg@gmail.com

Y. Huang, D.O. • P. Mancini, M.D. • S. Gruenbaum, M.D.
Department of Anesthesiology, Yale University School of Medicine,
333 Cedar Street, 208051, New Haven, CT 06520-8051, USA
e-mail: Yili.huang@yale.edu

A. Vadivelu, B.D.S., M.D.S.
Annoor Dental College and Hospital, Muvattupuzha, Kerala 686673, India
e-mail: Amarvadivelu@gmail.com

S. Dabu-Bondoc, M.D.
Department of Anesthesiology, Yale University School of Medicine,
333 Cedar Street, 208051, New Haven, CT 06520-8051, USA

Haven Hospital, 333 Cedar Street, 208051, New Haven, CT 06520-8051, USA
e-mail: Susan.Dabu-Bondoc@yale.edu

Finally, the neurobiology and key aspects of neuropathic orofacial pain and pain due to temporomandibular dysfunction, two of the most perplexing orofacial syndromes, are also discussed.

Primary Afferent Nociceptor

There are three different types of primary peripheral afferents. Aβ fibers are myelinated and thick, allowing the Aβ fibers to be the fastest conducting fibers. Aδ fibers have thinner, myelinated axons and are slower than Aβ fibers. Finally, C fibers are the thinnest and unmyelinated, making C fibers the slowest fibers for conductance [3].

The orofacial region is mainly innervated by the trigeminal nerve, whose primary afferent cell bodies rest within the trigeminal ganglion. These neurons generally possess type Aδ or C fibers [4]. While the fast type Aβ fibers are activated via light touch and pressure, the slower Aδ and C fibers of the trigeminal region, collectively termed nociceptors, respond to pain. The activation of these two types of nociceptors is associated with substantial release of substance P, which modulates pain sensitivity by the activation of neurokinin-1 receptors [5].

These nociceptors can be further subdivided into mechanonociceptors (sensitive to mechanical stimuli), thermo-nociceptors (sensitive to heat or cold), and chemo-nociceptors (sensitive to chemicals). The thermo-nociceptors are found to possess vanilloid receptor 1-like receptors that contribute to the pain caused by extreme temperatures [6]. Similarly, the mechanoreceptors found in the root pulp are lined with epithelial Na^+ channels that are responsible for sharp pain induced by liquid motion in the dentinal tubules [7].

Modulation to these nociceptors can also be mechanical or chemical in nature. Canine studies have demonstrated that the threshold for mechanonociception can be lower with periodontal inflammation and can thus increase sensitization [8]. This may be due to the hydrodynamic mechanism of inflammation in the noncompliant environment of the dentine-encased pulp, which increases the pressure on the pulp and thereby activates the nociceptors [9]. Furthermore, there is considerable peripheral and central modulation due to the many types of neuropeptides released during tissue damage and localized within the trigeminal ganglia. These peptides, such as substance P and calcitonin-related peptide, play a vital role in sensitizing the nociceptors leading to allodynia (pain to innocuous stimuli) and hyperalgesia (increased response to painful stimuli) [10].

Finally, unlike the spinal system, where damage of a peripheral nerve causes hypersensitivity to noxious stimuli of nearby skin, nerve damage and territorial hypersensitivity of the trigeminal spinal nucleus are much less predictable [11]. Transection of the inferior alveolar nerve induces hypersensitivity of the trigeminal neurons in the upper lip, outside the territory of the inferior alveolar nerve [12]. A possible explanation of this phenomenon may have to do with the uniquely different central relay of the trigeminal system.

Central Relay

In the brainstem, the primary afferent neurons terminate at the trigeminal spinal tract nucleus. This nucleus consists of three subnuclei: subnucleus oralis, subnucleus interpolaris, and subnucleus caudalis. The subnucleus caudalis serves as the main brainstem relay for nociception and is so structurally similar to the spinal dorsal horn, an important structure in spinal nociception, that it is often referred to as the trigeminal dorsal horn [13]. The subnucleus caudalis or the trigeminal dorsal horn is an important central structure for the modulation of nociception. Rat studies have suggested that disinhibition of the trigeminal subnucleus caudalis plays a major role in the appearance of allodynia after nerve damage [14]. Inflammation or trauma induces a central sensitization of the subnucleus caudalis through its afferent nociceptors via various physiologic and biochemical mechanisms such as ion channels, neurokinins, and N-methyl-D-aspartate (NMDA). This increases the excitability of the subnucleus and leads to allodynia, hyperalgesia, or even spontaneous pain. Conversely, descending inhibitory modulation, found mainly in the dorsomedial fields, occurs via behavioral or environmental triggers and can be a contributing mechanism in the efficacy of certain analgesics such as morphine and tricyclic antidepressants [15].

Although the other two subnuclei of the trigeminal spinal tract nucleus, the subnucleus oralis and subnucleus interpolaris, receive input from all three types of fiber, it receives a large proportion of input from fast-conducting Aβ fibers. This makes these subnuclei very versatile. Central neurons within these subnuclei can be further classified into nociceptive specific neurons, which are only Aδ and C fibers responding only to noxious stimuli, or wide dynamic range neurons, consisting of all three fiber types and responding to noxious and innocuous stimuli [16]. Deep pain is attributed to the convergence of different types of receptors into a central nociceptive neuron; the complexity of the convergences leads to misinterpretation of the original sensation, which contributes to hyperalgesia or allodynia [17]. Additional studies also indicate that the transition zone between the subnuclei caudalis and the subnuclei interpolaris also plays a role in the central processing of deep orofacial nociception [18].

Orofacial sensation continues up its path from the brainstem through the thalamus on its way to the cortex. Nociceptive specific neurons and wide dynamic range neurons are found scattered throughout the thalamus including the posterior nucleus, ventrobasal complex or ventral posterior nucleus, and intralaminar nucleus. The posterior nucleus is responsible for classifying a stimulus as pain, the ventrobasal complex or the ventral posterior nucleus localizes the pain to a region, and the intralaminar nucleus provides an affective and motivational dimension to the pain. In other words, the lateral thalamus projects to the somatosensory cerebral cortex to pinpoint the pain, while the medial thalamus projects to other areas such as the cingulate gyrus and hypothalamus to associate the pain with the proper emotions [19].

Biochemical Influences

Biochemical influences play a large role in the transmission and modulation of orofacial pain. Recent studies have focused on various biochemical neuroactive substances and proteins such as nitric oxide (NO), nicotinamide adenine dinucleotide phosphate-diaphorase (NADPH), GABA, glycine, and c-Fos and their roles in orofacial pain modulation.

Neurons within the subnucleus oralis and subnucleus caudalis produce nitric oxide, a substance that increases intracellular cyclic guanosine monophosphate levels to work as both an endothelial relaxing factor as well as a neurotransmitter [20]. Increased levels of nitric oxide have been associated with neuropathic pain associated with NMDA receptor stimulation [21]. Surprisingly, while NO is also associated with the maintenance of chronic pain, it has no association to the initiation of acute pain [22].

NADPH is found within the same neurons that produce NO as well as within neurons that produce GABA and glycine in the spinal dorsal horn. It is also co-localized with calbindin D and calretinin within the subnucleus oralis. These neurons project to the trigeminal motor nucleus and are involved with the modulation of the orofacial sensorimotor reflex. This explains the early appearance of subnucleus oralis NADPH during fetal development. This allows the human fetus to respond to facial stimuli as early as during the 7th week of gestation, long before the cerebral cortex has developed any motion controlling ability [23].

c-Fos is a complex DNA-binding protein that acts at the promoter region of a few neurotransmitter genes including encephalin, dynorphin, and cholecystokinin [24]. Its effect on nociception can vary greatly. Like the associated neurotransmitter dynorphin, the presence of c-Fos can contribute to antinociception through the Kappa-opioid receptor [25]. Conversely, this action is complicated by c-Fos' ability to contribute to the neuro-inflammatory cascade that aids in creating a hyperalgesic state.

Like c-Fos and dynorphins, GABA also has a complicated response to nociception. GABA is an inhibitory neurotransmitter that acts mainly in the central nervous system with two different receptors: GABA(A), which involves Cl channel conductance, and GABA(B), which involves cGMP-coupled regulation of Ca^+ and K^+ conductance.

GABA(A) receptor antagonism increases the sensation of innocuous stimuli within the trigeminal sensory nuclei [26]. This is mainly due to its effects on the segmental sites [27]. In stark contrast, GABAergic disinhibition on the supraspinal sites, such as the nucleus raphe or the periaqueductal grey, decreases the effect of high-intensity noxious stimuli. The systemic effect of the GABA(A) receptors, therefore, is to equilibrate sensation towards a medium.

Baclofen is an antispasmodic that works as a GABA(B) receptor agonist. As stated above, GABA(B) receptors, located in the Aδ and C fibers, decrease excitatory transmission via decreased Ca^+ influx and increased K^+ currents. Baclofen, via its agonism of the GABA(B) receptors, has been found to aid in decreasing nociceptive response in both the trigeminal as well as the spinal systems [28].

There are a plethora of biochemical influences that moderate the trigeminal sensory system. They combine to moderate nociception, but a dysfunction or a misbalance of these substances can lead to pathologic orofacial pain processes as seen in neuropathic pain or temporomandibular disorders (TMD).

Neuropathic Orofacial Pain

The trigeminal system is relatively insulated from neuropathic pain. Compared with the spinal system, there is a lower disposition to and quicker recovery from neuropathic pain [29]. This, however, does not make it immune to neurologic pain states. Three orofacial pain conditions that must be considered are trigeminal neuropathic pain, atypical facial pain, and progression into chronic pain.

Neuropathic orofacial pain can be classified into four types: pain associated with nerve damage, insidious pain generally from an organic source such as a neoplasm, vascular pain associated with migraines, and burning, constant pain without any inciting event [30]. Trigeminal neuropathic pain is an example of the first type as there is often evidence of a trigeminal nerve lesion, although there may also be a vascular etiology to this condition [31]. Centrally, this condition may also be by multiple sclerosis. Neuropathic orofacial pain usually presents with sensory symptoms such as burning pain, allodynia, and hyperalgesia that are well localized with defined trigger zones.

In contrast to trigeminal neuropathic pain, atypical facial pain really lacks a significant cause and generally presents with constant, burning, deep, and poorly localized pain. In fact, the International Headache Society classifies atypical facial pain as "Facial Pain Not Fulfilling Other Criteria." While it is suggested that atypical facial pain may be caused by hyperactive central neuronal activity due to damage to the primary afferent neurons, it is likely that atypical facial pain is also a combination of different clinical entities as a result of biological and psychological contributions [32]. In addition, phantom tooth pain, a type of atypical facial pain, has been associated with a neurovascular etiology [33]. There is a high correlation of atypical facial pain with psychological disorders, but there is often a question of whether the pain is the cause or rather the effect of these disorders. Studies have found that a large percentage of patients also suffer from clinical depression and had histories of abuse. This suggests that the pain may in fact be an effect of the prior psychological insults [34].

Neuropathic orofacial pain may eventually persist into a chronic pain state following neuronal injury. This is because certain initially insensitive mechanonociceptors may become sensitized following injury leading to hyperalgesia and allodynia. Central sensitization also plays a vital role. This concept suggests that an increased sensitivity of central pain signaling causes an elevated responsiveness to and reception of the initial sensation. This can help explain phantom limb syndromes as well as hyperalgesia and allodynia associated with neuronal and tissue damage [35].

Temporomandibular Joint Disorders

Another prominent orofacial pain pathology is classified as TMD. These are pain conditions related to the jaw muscles and the temporomandibular joint (TMJ) and are major cause of non-dental orofacial pain [36]. The symptoms include deep and diffuse pain associated with jaw motion, ear pain, TMJ clicking, and limited jaw opening.

Although the pathophysiology of TMD pain is unclear, it is associated with psychologic factors [37]. Interestingly, TMD also seems to be associated with irritable bowel syndrome, another pain syndrome with a very different anatomic location. These associations suggest that chronic pain conditions such as TMD are related via a central mechanism, regardless of the site of pain [38]. Recent studies have also suggested that there are genetic risk factors associated with TMD symptomatology, especially those related to estrogen [39]. Estrogen status and chronic inflammation, through a common mitogen-activated protein kinase/extracellular regulated kinase, enhance central nociception in TMD [40].

Conclusion

From the primary afferent nociceptors to the somatosensory cerebral cortex, the neurobiology of orofacial pain is a complex and dynamic process, with ongoing biochemical modulation of orofacial pain and TMD. There are often genetic, psychological, and social components to the development of orofacial pain, and its neurobiology is best examined with a multidisciplinary approach.

Acknowledgements The authors would like to thank Nirmal Kumar Vadivelu Amarender and Gopal Kodumudi and Vijay Kodumudi for their help in the preparation of this manuscript.

Conflict of Interest None declared.

References

1. Stewart WF, Ricci JA, Chee E, Morganstein D, Lipton R. Lost productive time and cost due to common pain conditions in the US workforce. JAMA. 2003;290(18):2443–54.
2. Sessle BJ, Baad-Hansen L, Svennsson P. Orofacial pain. In: Lynch ME, Craig KD, Peng PWH, editors. Clinical pain management: a practical guide. 1st ed. Hoboken, NJ: Blackwell; 2011.
3. Hunt CC. Relation of function to diameter in afferent fibers of muscle nerves. J Gen Physiol. 1954;38(1):117–31. PMID: 13192320.
4. Dubner R, Sessle BJ, Storey AT. The neural basis of oral and facial function. New York: Plenum; 1978.
5. Jessell TM. Substance P in nociceptive sensory neurons. Ciba Found Symp. 1982;91:225–48.
6. Ichikawa H, Sugimoto T. Vanilloid receptor 1-like receptor-immunoreactive primary sensory neurons in the rat trigeminal nervous system. Neuroscience. 2000;101(3):719–25.

7. Ichikawa H, Fukuda T, Terayama R, Yamaai T, Kuboki T, Sugimoto T. Immunohistochemical localization of gamma and beta subunits of epithelial Na+ channel in the rat molar tooth pulp. Brain Res. 2005;1065(1–2):138–41. Epub 2005 Nov 17.
8. Matsumoto H. [Effects of pulpal inflammation on the activities of periodontal mechanoreceptive afferent fibers]. Kokubyo Gakkai Zasshi. 2010;77(2):115–20. Japanese.
9. Mathews B, Sessle BJ. Peripheral mechanisms of orofacial pain. In: Sessle BJ, Lavigne GL, Lund JP, et al., editors. Orofacial pain. 2nd ed. Chicago, IL: Quintessence; 2008. p. 27–43.
10. Meyer RA, Ringkamp M, Campbell JN, et al. Peripheral mechanisms of cutaneous nociception. In: McMahon SB, Koltzenburg M, editors. Wall and Melzacks textbook of pain. 5th ed. Amsterdam: Elsevier; 2006. p. 3–34.
11. Sugimoto T, Ichikawa H, Hijiya H, Mitani S, Nakago T. c-Fos expression by dorsal horn neurons chronically deafferented by peripheral nerve section in response to spared, somatotopically inappropriate nociceptive primary input. Brain Res. 1993;621(1):161–6.
12. Nomura H, Ogawa A, Tashiro A, Morimoto T, Hu JW, Iwata K. Induction of Fos protein-like immunoreactivity in the trigeminal spinal nucleus caudalis and upper cervical cord following noxious and non-noxious mechanical stimulation of the whisker pad of the rat with an inferior alveolar nerve transection. Pain. 2002;95(3):225–38.
13. Gobel S, Bennett GJ, Allen B, Humphrey E, Seltzer Z, Abdelmoumene M, Hayashi H, Hoffert MJ. Synaptic connectivity of substantia gelatinosa neurons with reference to potential termination site of descending axons. In: Sjolund B, Bjorkland A, editors. Brain stem control of spinal mechanisms. New York: Elsevier/North Holland; 1982.
14. Martin YB, Malmierca E, Avendaño C, Nuñez A. Neuronal disinhibition in the trigeminal nucleus caudalis in a model of chronic neuropathic pain. Eur J Neurosci. 2010;32(3): 399–408.
15. Gojyo F, Sugiyo S, Kuroda R, Kawabata A, Varathan V, Shigenaga Y, Takemura M. Effects of somatosensory cortical stimulation on expression of c-Fos in rat medullary dorsal horn in response to formalin-induced noxious stimulation. J Neurosci Res. 2002;68(4):479–88.
16. Tenenbaum HC, Mock D, Gordon AS, Goldberg MB, Grossi ML, Locker D, Davis KD. Sensory and affective components of orofacial pain: is it all in your brain? Crit Rev Oral Biol Med. 2001;12(6):455–68.
17. Ness TJ, Gebhart GF. Visceral pain: a review of experimental studies. Pain. 1990;41(2):167–234.
18. Shimizu K, Guo W, Wang H, Zou S, LaGraize SC, Iwata K, Wei F, Dubner R, Ren K. Differential involvement of trigeminal transition zone and laminated subnucleus caudalis in orofacial deep and cutaneous hyperalgesia: the effects of interleukin-10 and glial inhibitors. Mol Pain. 2009;5:75.
19. Willis WD. Nociceptive functions of thalamic neurons. In: Sterlade M, Jones EG, McCormick DA, editors. Thalamus. Oxford: Elsevier Science; 1997.
20. Bredt DS, Glatt CE, Hwang PM, Fotuhi M, Dawson TM, Snyder SH. Nitric oxide synthase protein and mRNA are discretely localized in neuronal populations of the mammalian CNS together with NADPH diaphorase. Neuron. 1991;7(4):615–24.
21. Laing I, Todd AJ, Heizmann CW, Schmidt HH. Subpopulations of GABAergic neurons in laminae I-III of rat spinal dorsal horn defined by coexistence with classical transmitters, peptides, nitric oxide synthase or parvalbumin. Neuroscience. 1994;61(1):123–32.
22. Yonehara N, Takemura M, Yoshimura M, Iwase K, Seo HG, Taniguchi N, Shigenaga Y. Nitric oxide in the rat spinal cord in Freund's adjuvant-induced hyperalgesia. Jpn J Pharmacol. 1997;75(4):327–35.
23. Takemura M, Wakisaka S, Iwase K, Yabuta NH, Nakagawa S, Chen K, Bae YC, Yoshida A, Shigenaga Y. NADPH-diaphorase in the developing rat: lower brainstem and cervical spinal cord, with special reference to the trigemino-solitary complex. J Comp Neurol. 1996;365(4):511–25.
24. Dubner R, Ruda MA. Activity-dependent neuronal plasticity following tissue injury and inflammation. Trends Neurosci. 1992;15(3):96–103. Review.
25. Millan MJ. Multiple opioid systems and pain. Pain. 1986;27(3):303–47.
26. Takemura M, Shimada T, Shigenaga Y. GABA(A) receptor-mediated effects on expression of c-Fos in rat trigeminal nucleus following high- and low-intensity afferent stimulation. Neuroscience. 2000;98(2):325–32.

27. Hwang JH, Yaksh TL. The effect of spinal GABA receptor agonists on tactile allodynia in a surgically-induced neuropathic pain model in the rat. Pain. 1997;70(1):15–22.
28. Price GW, Wilkin GP, Turnbull MJ, Bowery NG. Are baclofen-sensitive GABAB receptors present on primary afferent terminals of the spinal cord? Nature. 1984;307(5946):71–4.
29. Svensson P, Baad-Hansen L. Facial pain. In: Wilson P, Watson PJ, Haythornthwaite JA, et al., editors. Clinical pain management: chronic pain. 2nd ed. Cornwall: Hodder Arnold; 2008. p. 467–83.
30. Loeser JD. Tic douloureux and atypical facial pain. In: Wall PD, Melzack R, editors. Textbook of pain. Edinburgh: Churchill Livingstone; 1994. p. 699–710.
31. Benoliel R, Sharav Y. Chronic orofacial pain. Curr Pain Headache Rep. 2010;14(1):33–40.
32. Sessle BJ. Neurobiology of facial and dental pain. In: Sarnat BC, Laskin DM, editors. The temporomandibular joint: a biological basis for clinical practice. Philadelphia: WB Saunders; 1992. p. 124–42.
33. Rees RT, Harris M. Atypical odontalgia. Br J Oral Surg. 1979;16(3):212–8.
34. Riley 3rd JL, Robinson ME, Kvaal SA, Gremillion HA. Effects of physical and sexual abuse in facial pain: direct or mediated? Cranio. 1998;16(4):259–66.
35. Davis KD, Kiss ZH, Luo L, Tasker RR, Lozano AM, Dostrovsky JO. Phantom sensations generated by thalamic microstimulation. Nature. 1998;391(6665):385–7.
36. Bell WE. Orofacial pains: classification, diagnosis, management. 4th ed. Chicago: Year Book Medical Publishers; 1989.
37. Fricton JR, Olsen T. Predictors of outcome for treatment of temporomandibular disorders. J Orofac Pain. 1996;10(1):54–65.
38. Aaron LA, Burke MM, Buchwald D. Overlapping conditions among patients with chronic fatigue syndrome, fibromyalgia, and temporomandibular disorder. Arch Intern Med. 2000;160(2):221–7.
39. Kim BS, Kim YK, Yun PY, Lee E, Bae J. The effects of estrogen receptor α polymorphism on the prevalence of symptomatic temporomandibular disorders. J Oral Maxillofac Surg. 2010;68(12):2975–9. Epub 2010.
40. Tashiro A, Okamoto K, Bereiter DA. Chronic inflammation and estradiol interact through MAPK activation to affect TMJ nociceptive processing by trigeminal caudalis neurons. Neuroscience. 2009;164(4):1813–20. Epub 2009.

Chapter 2
Oral Health-Related Quality of Life and Facial Pain

Amarender Vadivelu

Introduction

Orofacial pain, as a specific sensory modality, has four tangible components: perceptual, emotional, visceral, and referral component. Pain can lead to tissue damage. Prevention of tissue damage becomes an overriding concern in the management of orofacial pain. Other states related to facial pain include anxiety, fear, stress, panic, and depression. These states affect the expression of pain [1] and hence the quality of life. Quality of life has been defined as a broad multidimensional concept that includes subjective evaluations of both positive and negative aspects of life. Health, financial status, divorce, bereavement, and other life events impact the quality of life. Disease and infirmity can take their toll by affecting normal physiological functions and hindering daily activities of living. The ability to perform day to day activities liking walking, driving and perception of the sense of smell, touch and taste are crucial to optimal quality of life.

The aforementioned activities and perceptions are altered by disease and need prompt attention. A disorder in question is anosmia: How anosmia leads to loss of olfactory control, which in turn can hinder the ability to sense the multitude of flavors present in food, which is of paramount importance in enjoying a good meal? Maxillofacial injuries apart from causing pain can damage nerves leading to paresis of the tongue with resultant loss of function. It is no exaggeration to state that pain can cause a functional deficit and derange the quality of life.

Health-related quality of life at its best would be a cherished end point for a health care practitioner and has been advocated as a supplemental measure for incorporation in public health policy in addition to traditional measures like statistics related to mortality and morbidity.

A. Vadivelu, B.D.S., M.D.S. (✉)
Annoor Dental College and Hospital, Muvattupuzha, Kerala 686673, India
e-mail: Amarvadivelu@gmail.com

General Health- and Oral Health-Related Quality of Life

Intractable facial pain, which includes orofacial and craniofacial pain, can affect the general well-being of the individual and his or her ability to perform daily chores in a facile manner. This in turn may translate to lost man-hours and a drop in wages and, as a consequence, affect the self-esteem of an individual. This cascading effect resulting from facial pain can lead to tissue damage as well as peripheral and central nervous system sensitization, all of which present a formidable challenge to the treating pain physician. Thus oral health-related quality of life (OHRQoL) should not be viewed in isolation for treatment planning but as an integral part of sound functional overall health.

Facial Disorders, Facial Pain, and OHRQoL

A review of some of the clinical conditions causing pain and affecting the OHRQoL is in order to appreciate the burden of disease on hand.

Jaw Fractures

Fractured jaws are treated with reduction and immobilization using intermaxillary fixation by wires binding the upper and lower teeth together for a period ranging from 6 to 8 weeks. This will entail a transient loss of chewing ability and lead to stiffness and pain in the affected muscles. The patient has to use a feeding cup with a tube placed in the buccal vestibule to enable suction of fluid/puree diet for the period of treatment followed by oral rehabilitation exercises.

Temporomandibular Disorders

The jaw joint can be affected by a host of clinical problems impacting OHRQoL. Subluxation and early-morning locking of the jaws due to intracapsular disorders, clicking sounds, or dislocation of the mandible due to excessive yawning can result in pain and inability to chew food. These disorders can cause varying degrees of temporomandibular dysfunction, pain muscle spasm, and impairment of OHRQoL.

Stroke and OHRQoL

Cerebrovascular accidents can cause distorted facial features, dysregulation of swallowing, and facial paralysis. The OHRQoL is affected to an advanced degree by considerable neurological deficit. Feeding of patients with a neurological deficit of impaired swallowing has to be done with a nasogastric tube in place for extended time periods.

Migraine and OHRQoL

Migraine can be intractable and can cause bouts of prolonged severe pain culminating in absence from work. The condition requires reassurance and pharmacotherapy.

Cleft Lip and Palate

These are congenital defects and impair OHRQoL from infancy through adulthood. The psychological impact of this disorder is tremendous. The biopsychosocial model integrating biologic, psychologic, and social components as propounded by Dworkin Von Korff and LeResche in 1992 has a huge bearing in chronic pain and disorders like cleft lip and palate [2]. The infant needs a feeding plate due to oronasal incompetence. Plastic surgery may be required to correct the cleft, which in turn leads to scarring and mal development of the palate. Orthodontic treatment is also required. It has been stated that individuals with craniofacial anomalies have structurally different faces from normal individuals [3]; this would have a definite bearing on OHRQoL from the patient's perspective, and they may have to be judged on a different aesthetic scale [4].

Ankyloglossia

Ankyloglossia or tongue tie is a distressing condition and needs surgical correction. Compromised movement of the tongue leads to lisping in speech. The emotional dimension of this problem is reflected in an aberrant OHRQoL.

Ageusia

Loss of taste sensation can hamper perceiving the taste sensations of sweet, salty, bitter, and sour. This could also be an occupational hazard in wine tasters and tea tasters if for any reason they are affected by nerve injuries to the face.

Radiotherapy and Surgery for Oral and Nasal Cancer

Treatment of oral cancer often requires radiotherapy which can lead to impaired OHRQoL such as pain in radiation mucositis, xerostomia, and radiation caries. Patients with nasal cancer need a nasal prosthesis after ablative surgery.

Indices for Oral Health-Related Quality of Life

Notable indices are the oral health impact profile (OHIP Slade and Spencer 1994) [5] and the dental aesthetic index [6].

The OHIP is a questionnaire for adults and assesses oral function, pain, social disability, and handicap. The index is widely used and has the potential for translation into different languages to assess oral health quality of life parameters in patients whose native language is not English.

Other indices are the abridged version of the OHIP known as OHIP-14 and OHIP-20; UK oral health related quality of life measure (OHQoL-UK); oral impacts on daily performances (OIDP); Geriatric (General) Oral Health Assessment Index (GOHAI); Child Oral Health Quality of Life Questionnaire (COHQOL); and Orthogenetic Quality of Life Questionnaire (OQoLQ).

The dental aesthetic index, although intended to measure malocclusion, has the elements of malocclusion, social dimension, and psychological dimension built into the index. The index demonstrates the importance of social appearance as an indicator of self-esteem.

Need for Qualitative Research

Qualitative research needs to be conducted across pain settings to gather data on OHRQoL to set targets for correcting oral health disparities and alleviation of facial pain. In addition research aids in identifying populations at risk to assist in formulating public health policies and allocating financial outlays in the health budget to carry out tangible oral health initiatives. Governments of various countries can take a cue from Bhutan who has incorporated "Gross National Happiness" as a quality-of-life measure for progress. The instruments to measure OHRQoL can be tailored to ascertain "within-subject" changes in clinical studies by incorporating disease-specific items in the questionnaire.

Recommendations on Future of Dental Education

Inglehart has cited a stellar recommendation on the future of dental education enunciated by a committee of the Institute of Medicine [7]. These include educating oral health professionals on the perspective of true patient-centered care, sensitivity to transcultural health issues, and perception of oral health in the context of patients' overall health.

Summary

The potential of facial pain to cause tissue damage and its negative influence on OHRQoL has been given credence in this commentary. An overview of various clinical disorders with pain as a cardinal sign has been presented. Future training of dental professionals should include sensitivity to transcultural issues and see oral health as an integral part of general well-being. Alleviation of pain is an important goal in the overall treatment plan of mouth rehabilitation.

In essence, optimal quality of life is the cherished aspiration of every individual. This behooves the health care practitioner to make a paradigm shift in health care delivery to incorporate sound quality of life as an end point in the therapeutic protocol.

Acknowledgement None declared.

Conflict of Interest None declared.

References

1. Keefe FJ, Lumley M, Anderson T, Lynch T, Carson KL. Pain and emotion: new research directions. J Clin Psychol. 2001;57:587–607.
2. Dworkin SF, Von Korff M, LeResche L. Epidemiologic studies of chronic pain: a dynamic-ecologic perspective. Ann Behav Med. 1992;14:3–11.
3. Eder R. Craniofacial anomalies: psychological perspectives. New York: Springer; 1995.
4. Giddon DB, Anderson NK. The oral and craniofacial area and interpersonal attraction. In: Mostofsky DI, Forgione AG, Giddon DB, editors. Behavioral dentistry. Iowa: Blackwell Munksgaard; 2006. p. 3–17.
5. Slade GD, Spencer AJ. Development and evaluation of the oral health impact profile. Community Dent Health. 1994;11:3–11.
6. Jenny J, Cons NC, Kohout FJ. Comparison of SASOC, a measure of dental aesthetics, with three orthodontic indices and orthodontist judgment. Community Dent Oral Epidemiol. 1983;11:236–41.
7. Inglehart MR. Oral health and quality of life. In: Mostofsky DI, Forgione AG, Giddon DB, editors. Behavioral dentistry. Iowa: Blackwell Munksgaard; 2006. p. 19–28.

Chapter 3
Classification and Epidemiology of Orofacial Pain

Suhas Setty and Jamil David

Introduction

There are several classification schemes that have been reported in the literature. The majority are based on either the structures involved or the symptoms. Some classifications are based on cluster analysis of pain conditions, and some are based on diagnostic criteria. A few of the popular known ones include:

- International association for the study of pain (IASP) [1]
- Research diagnostic criteria for temporomandibular diseases (RDC/TMD) [2]
- American academy of orofacial pain guidelines [3]
- ICD10—G 50.0 disorders of trigeminal nerve [4]

Classification systems have evolved over time from a simple one-dimensional location-based system to multidimensional/multiaxial systems [1, 2, 5]. Basic need to develop a classification would be to distinguish one entity from another, in other words make a "differential diagnosis," which would eventually help a clinician in decision making regarding identification of the disease process as well as prognosis and treatment planning. Classification systems for orofacial pain published to date have not been able to provide a clear allocation of the disease to the category because of the numerous overlapping pathophysiology as well as symptomatology.

In this chapter a simple and broad classification for orofacial pain conditions is proposed, and epidemiology for each of the classifications is described as reported in various literatures.

S. Setty, B.D.S., M.D.S. (✉)
Department of Oral Medicine and Radiology, Sri Siddhartha Dental College, Tumkur, India
e-mail: suhassetty@gmail.com

J. David, B.D.S., M.Sc., Ph.D.
Department of Health Services Research, University of Liverpool, Liverpool, UK

Classification

A broad classification for clinically determined orofacial pain can be categorized as tooth related and non-tooth related; they could be further subclassified as shown in Table 3.1.

Facial pain can also be classified as peripheral or central; this of course will be a very primitive method; commonly, facial pain symptoms are caused by local factors, usually in the oral cavity or adjacent structures with teeth and temporomandibular joints being the major sources of peripheral facial pain. Central facial pain is always secondary to intracranial pathology, such as neoplasms, vascular compression, and other idiopathic phenomena.

Epidemiology of Orofacial Pain

Accurate incidence estimates for facial pain in the general population are scant; prevalence of up to 26 % has been reported [6]. Presented below is the epidemiology for different causes of orofacial pain.

Table 3.1 Classification based on clinical presentation of orofacial pain

1. Tooth related
    a. Pulpal
        i   Dentinal hypersensitivity resulting from
            - Caries
            - Wasting disease
        ii Pulp disease (reversible and irreversible pulpitis) resulting from
            - Caries
            - Trauma
    b. Pathology in periapical region—acute abscess
    c. Gum/periodontal diseases
    d. Cracked tooth syndrome
2. Non-tooth related
    a. Musculoskeletal—temporomandibular diseases (TMD)
    b. Neuralgias and neuropathic
        i   Trigeminal, glossopharyngeal, sphenopalatine
        ii Post injury
        iii Postherpetic neuralgia, burning mouth syndrome
    c. Idiopathic orofacial pain
    d. Mucosal—traumatic, immunologic, infective, erosive, ulcerative, and vesiculobullous lesions
    e. Psychosomatic
    f. Sinonasal
    g. Headaches—migraine, tension type, brain tumors, and aneurysms
    h. Salivary gland diseases—sialadenitis, sialolithiasis
    i. Cardiac toothache

Tooth-Related Orofacial Pain

Toothache (dental pain) is the most common amongst the causes of pain symptoms in the mouth, and this invariably affects quality of life. Epidemiological studies about dental pain are few, and hence it is difficult to infer its patterns [7, 8]. Dental pain is highly prevalent among children and is consistently associated with population levels of caries experience, the association being most apparent in lower socioeconomic groups with reduced access to care [9–11]. Tooth-related pain is strongly correlated with untreated dental disease (dental decay); in addition, fractured teeth and exposed dentin due to attrition, erosion, and abrasion may also cause pain. Impacted third molars also cause pain; 23 % of partially erupted impacted third molars develop pain symptoms compared to 10 % of unerupted [12]. It is also reported that tooth-related disease and pain in children are inversely associated with educational levels of parents [13, 14] as well as educational levels of individuals [15, 16]. Gender association of toothache is difficult to conclude, with the association being inconsistent [17].

Cracked or fractured tooth may be the reason for unexplained pain in a vital, amalgam-restored tooth. Cracked teeth are usually found in the molars with higher incidence in mandibular molars [18]. They are common in the fourth decade of life [18, 19] and in teeth with restorations involving the marginal ridges [20]. Among patients suffering from gum/periodontal diseases pain levels are minimum in those with gingivitis (6 %) and gradually increase as the disease progresses, manifesting periodontal pockets/loss of attachment (25 %) [21, 22].

Acute periapical abscess as well as acute exacerbation of chronic periapical abscess resulting as a sequel of pulp necrosis invariably induce pain; pain may or may not be accompanied by swelling [23, 24].

Non-tooth-Related Orofacial Pain

Temporomandibular Disorders and Orofacial Pain

Temporomandibular disorders (TMD) represent clusters of related disorders in the masticatory system. They are characterized by pain in the temporomandibular joint (TMJ) and/or pain in the preauricular area or muscles of mastication and may or may not be accompanied by TMJ sounds and/or deviations/restrictions in the mandibular range of movement. TMD are a major cause of non-dental pain in the orofacial region, and oral health-related quality of life is markedly impaired in these patients [25]. There is no strong association of gender for TMD [26]; however, it is found that a higher proportion of women seek treatment [27]. TMD are more common among patients with impaired general health [28, 29]. In otherwise healthy population it is a prevalent disease. It is very rare among children less than 5 years [30] and is evident in teenagers with a prevalence of up to 10.5 % [30–32]. Increasing age, general health factors, and oral parafunctions are generally associated with TMD symptoms and signs. No clear relationship has been established between occlusal alterations and TMJ disease [32, 33]. Parafunctional habits and bruxism are considered risk factors of TMD [34] with odds ratio of up to 4.8 [32]. Stress is considered a major component for TMD [35]. Post-traumatic stress disorder patients are at increased risk for the development of TMD symptoms [36]. A substantial proportion of TMD patients have been found to be depressed and experience moderate to severe somatization [37]. Fifty-six percent of patients suffering from headaches, which include migraine, tension-type headache, and chronic daily headache, show at least one sign of TMD [38, 39]. A high prevalence of TMD has been noticed among obstructive sleep apnea patients [40]. Myofascial pain-associated TMD forms about 10.5 % of TMD [41]. Also, non-occlusion (posterior teeth, at least one side) and an open bite have been found to increase the risk of myofascial pain [42].

Neuralgias and Neuropathic Orofacial Pain

Prevalence of trigeminal neuralgia (TN) is low with an incidence range of about 4 to 5/100,000/year [43, 44] and increases with advancing age [44, 45]. It is more common among women (female:male = 3:2) [43]. TN pain is more predominant on the right side [45], but the difference is not statistically significant [44]. It has been hypothesized that smaller size of foramen rotundum and ovale on the right side are the causes of such presentation [46]. TN also manifests in up to 6 % of multiple sclerosis patients [47].

Glossopharyngeal neuralgia (GN) has an incidence of 0.7/100,000/year, and epidemiological studies have shown it to be less severe than previously thought [44, 48].

Sphenopalatine neuralgia is a rare craniofacial pain syndrome with higher prevalence in women [49, 50]. Chronic pain manifesting as varying degrees of paraesthesia, allodynia, or hyperalgesia is often a symptom following injury to lingual as well as inferior alveolar nerves [51]. Neuropathic orofacial pain as a result of deafferentation in trigeminal nerve fibers following endodontic and minor oral surgical procedures has also been reported in literature [52]. However, there are no true estimates available on its incidence and prevalence. Postherpetic neuralgia (PHN) is one of the long-term complications associated with herpes zoster infection and has a comparable incidence to idiopathic TN [44]. It has been estimated that up to 30 % of patients suffering from herpes zoster infection develop PHN, and it increases with increase in age [53]. As with TN, PHN is common among women [54]. Burning mouth syndrome is characterized by an oral burning sensation in the tongue or other oral mucous membrane in the absence of any clinical abnormal findings. It frequently affects middle-aged and aged women, with prevalence rates ranging from 0.6 to 12.22 % [55, 56].

Table 3.2 Prevalence of mucosal lesions

Mucosal lesion	Prevalence
Oral lichen planus	0.5–2.2 % of the population [62]
Pemphigus vulgaris	0.1–0.5 patients per 10^5 population per year [63]
Recurrent aphthous ulcers	5–60 % of population [64]
Radiation-induced mucositis	75 % of treated population [65]
Cancer chemotherapy-induced mucositis	40–70 % of treated population [65]
Mucositis in hemopoietic stem cell transplantation	75–99 % of treated population [65]

Idiopathic Orofacial Pain

Atypical facial pain, stomatodynia, atypical odontalgia, and some forms of masticatory muscle and temporomandibular joint disorders all seem to belong to the same group of idiopathic orofacial pain illnesses [57]. It is seen commonly in women and in the fourth decade of life. It is noticed in up to 6 % of patients undergoing endodontic treatment [58]. True prevalence or incidence rates of idiopathic orofacial pain have not been reported in literature.

Painful Oral Mucosal Lesions

Oral mucosal lesions are highly prevalent (Table 3.2), and painful oral ulcers are one of the main presenting symptoms of acute as well as chronic oral mucosal lesions (traumatic, infective, or immunologic) [59, 60]. Lesion prevalence differs significantly by age, sex, race/ethnicity, general health, denture wearing, and tobacco use [61].

Psychosomatic Diseases and Orofacial Pain

Stress, anxiety, psychological, as well as psychiatric disorders contribute substantially to causing orofacial pains and manifest as muscle tenderness, vague pains, and associated sleep disorders with no identifiable source of pain [66, 67]. Coexisting stress/anxiety disorders have been identified in 7 % of the population reporting with new onset of chronic orofacial pain [68].

Sinonasal Diseases and Orofacial Pain

Orofacial pain can originate from diseases of the sinonasal complex; it is most common from maxillary sinus diseases where pain is experienced even in the upper molar teeth along with pain over antral and forehead region [69]. Prevalence rates of maxillary sinusitis in the general population of up to 5 % in Canadians [70] and 14 % in Americans [71] have been reported.

Salivary Gland Diseases and Orofacial Pain

Inflammation and pain are prominent features in nonneoplastic diseases of salivary glands. Chronic nonspecific type of sialadenitis is the most common (87 %) type of nonneoplastic disease of salivary gland [72].

Headache and Orofacial Pain

Headache is one of the most reported comorbidity states in patients with symptoms of orofacial pain [73]. An estimated 20 % of the general population suffers from headache; most common types are tension-type headache and migraine [74, 75]. Global prevalence for tension-type headache is found to be about 38 % and 10 % for migraine [76], and up to 9 % of patients with migraine present with facial pain [77]. Overall incidence rate for primary brain tumors in the United States is 13.8/100,000 [78], and facial pain can be a presenting feature for intracranial tumors [79, 80]. Aneurysms, intracranial as well as extracranial, can also present with pain in the orofacial region [81, 82].

Cardiac Toothache

Referred pain to the mandibular region due to cardiac ischemia/myocardial infarction is referred to as cardiac toothache and is characterized by pain provocation/aggravation by physical activity, pain relief at rest, and bilateralism [83] and might be the only presenting complaint [84]. Cardiac ischemia/myocardial infarction is a relatively prevalent disease in the general population, and incidence rate of up to 133/100,000/year has been reported in literature [85].

Conclusion

Orofacial pain is a prevalent symptom in the general population, and its impact in terms of diminishing quality of life is remarkable. Epidemiological data for subtypes of diseases producing pain in the orofacial region is not obtainable from present literature; hence, efforts to increase epidemiological studies should be made.

Essentially clinicians should be aware of the wide spectrum of diseases producing pain symptoms in the orofacial region so that they will be able to develop appropriate management strategies.

Acknowledgement None declared.

Conflict of Interest None declared.

References

1. Merskey H, Bogduk N, editors. Classification of chronic pain: descriptions of chronic pain syndromes and definitions of pain terms. 2nd ed. Seattle, WA: IASP Press; 1994.
2. Dworkin SF, LeResche L. Research diagnostic criteria for temporomandibular disorders: review, criteria, examinations and specifications, critique. J Craniomandib Disord. 1992;6:301–55.
3. De Leeuw R, editor. Orofacial pain: guidelines for assessment, diagnosis, and management, The American Academy of orofacial pain, American Academy of orofacial pain guidelines. 4th ed. Chicago: Quintessence Publishing Co, Inc.; 2008.
4. World Health Organization, International Statistical Classification of Diseases and Related Health Problems 10th Revision (ICD-10) Version for 2010 (http://apps.who.int/classifications/icd10/browse/2010/en#/G50-G59).
5. Sheffer CE, Deisinger JA, Cassisi JE, et al. A revised taxonomy of patients with chronic pain. Pain Med. 2007;8(4):312–25. PMID: 17610453.
6. Macfarlane TV, Blinkhorn AS, Davies RM, et al. Oro-facial pain in the community: prevalence and associated impact. Community Dent Oral Epidemiol. 2002;30(1):52–60. PMID:11918576.
7. Pau AK, Croucher R, Marcenes W. Prevalence estimates and associated factors for dental pain: a review. Oral Health Prev Dent. 2003;1(3):209–20. PMID:15641499.
8. Bastos JL, Gigante DP, Peres KG, et al. Social determinants of odontalgia in epidemiological studies: theoretical review and proposed conceptual model. Cien Saude Colet. 2007;12(6):1611–21. PMID:18813497.
9. Slade GD. Epidemiology of dental pain and dental caries among children and adolescents. Community Dent Health. 2001;18(4):219–27.
10. Cohen LA, Bonito AJ, Akin DR, Manski RJ, et al. Toothache pain: a comparison of visits to physicians, emergency departments and dentists. J Am Dent Assoc. 2008;139(9):1205–16.
11. Honkala E, Honkala S, Rimpelä A, et al. The trend and risk factors of perceived toothache among Finnish adolescents from 1977 to 1997. J Dent Res. 2001;80(9):1823–7.
12. Fernandes MJ, Ogden GR, Pitts NB, et al. Incidence of symptoms in previously symptom-free impacted lower third molars assessed in general dental practice. Br Dent J. 2009;207(5):E10. discussion 218–9.
13. Nomura LH, Bastos JL, Peres MA. Dental pain prevalence and association with dental caries and socioeconomic status in schoolchildren, Southern Brazil, 2002. Braz Oral Res. 2004;18(2):134–40.
14. Traebert J, Guimarães Ldo A, Durante EZ, et al. Low maternal schooling and severity of dental caries in Brazilian preschool children. Oral Health Prev Dent. 2009;7(1):39–45.
15. Borges CM, Cascaes AM, Fischer TK, et al. Dental and gingival pain and associated factors among Brazilian adolescents: an analysis of the Brazilian Oral Health Survey 2002–2003. Cad Saude Publica. 2008;24(8):1825–34.
16. Bastos JL, Gigante DP, Peres KG. Toothache prevalence and associated factors: a population based study in southern Brazil. Oral Dis. 2008;14(4):320–6.

17. Koopman JS, Dieleman JP, Huygen FJ, et al. Incidence of facial pain in the general population. Pain. 2009;147(1–3):122–7.
18. Lubisich EB, Hilton TJ, Ferracane J. Northwest precedent cracked teeth: a review of the literature. J Esthet Restor Dent. 2010;22(3):158–67.
19. Udoye CI, Jafarzadeh H. Cracked tooth syndrome: characteristics and distribution among adults in a Nigerian teaching hospital. J Endod. 2009;35(3):334–6.
20. Homewood CI. Cracked tooth syndrome–incidence, clinical findings and treatment. Aust Dent J. 1998;43(4):217–22.
21. Brennan DS, Spencer AJ, Roberts-Thomson KF. Quality of life and disability weights associated with periodontal disease. J Dent Res. 2007;86(8):713–7.
22. Cunha-Cruz J. Pain and discomfort are the main symptoms affecting the quality of life in periodontal disease. J Evid Based Dent Pract. 2008;8(2):101–2.
23. Campanelli CA, Walton RE, Williamson AE, et al. Vital signs of the emergency patient with pulpal necrosis and localized acute apical abscess. J Endod. 2008;34(3):264–7. Epub 2007 Dec 21.
24. Canadian Collaboration on Clinical Practice Guidelines in Dentistry (CCCD). Clinical practice guideline on treatment of acute apical abscess (AAA) in adults. Evid Based Dent. 2004;5(1):8.
25. John MT, Reissmann DR, Schierz O, et al. Oral health-related quality of life in patients with temporomandibular disorders. J Orofac Pain. 2007;21(1):46–54.
26. Mundt T, Mack F, Schwahn C, et al. Association between sociodemographic, behavioral, and medical conditions and signs of temporomandibular disorders across gender: results of the study of health in Pomerania (SHIP-0). Int J Prosthodont. 2008;21(2):141–8.
27. Bonjardim LR, Lopes-Filho RJ, Amado G, et al. Association between symptoms of temporomandibular disorders and gender, morphological occlusion, and psychological factors in a group of university students. Indian J Dent Res. 2009;20(2):190–4.
28. Burris JL, Evans DR, Carlson CR. Psychological correlates of medical comorbidities in patients with temporomandibular disorders. J Am Dent Assoc. 2010;141(1):22–31.
29. Johansson A, Unell L, Carlsson G, et al. Associations between social and general health factors and symptoms related to temporomandibular disorders and bruxism in a population of 50-year-old subjects. Acta Odontol Scand. 2004;62(4):231–7.
30. Köhler AA, Helkimo AN, Magnusson T, et al. Prevalence of symptoms and signs indicative of temporomandibular disorders in children and adolescents. A cross-sectional epidemiological investigation covering two decades. Eur Arch Paediatr Dent. 2009;10 Suppl 1:16–25.
31. Wu N, Hirsch C. Temporomandibular disorders in German and Chinese adolescents. J Orofac Orthop. 2010;71(3):187–98.
32. Poveda Roda R, Bagan JV, Díaz Fernández JM, et al. Review of temporomandibular joint pathology. Part I: classification, epidemiology and risk factors. Med Oral Patol Oral Cir Bucal. 2007;12(4):E292–8.
33. McNamara Jr JA, Seligman DA, Okeson JP. Occlusion, orthodontic treatment, and temporomandibular disorders: a review. J Orofac Pain. 1995;9(1):73–90.
34. Marklund S, Wänman A. Risk factors associated with incidence and persistence of signs and symptoms of temporomandibular disorders. Acta Odontol Scand. 2010;68(5):289–99.
35. Wahlund K. Temporomandibular disorders in adolescents. Epidemiological and methodological studies and a randomized controlled trial. Swed Dent J Suppl. 2003;164:2–64. inside front cover.
36. Uhac I, Kovac Z, Muhvić-Urek M, Kovacević D, et al. The prevalence of temporomandibular disorders in war veterans with post-traumatic stress disorder. Mil Med. 2006;171(11):1147–9.
37. Yap AU, Dworkin SF, Chua EK, et al. Prevalence of temporomandibular disorder subtypes, psychologic distress, and psychosocial dysfunction in Asian patients. J Orofac Pain. 2003;17(1):21–8.
38. Gonçalves DA, Bigal ME, Jales LC, et al. Headache and symptoms of temporomandibular disorder: an epidemiological study. Headache. 2010;50(2):231–41.

39. Ballegaard V, Thede-Schmidt-Hansen P, Svensson P, et al. Are headache and temporomandibular disorders related? A blinded study. Cephalalgia. 2008;28(8):832–41.
40. Cunali PA, Almeida FR, Santos CD, Valdrighi NY, et al. Prevalence of temporomandibular disorders in obstructive sleep apnea patients referred for oral appliance therapy. J Orofac Pain. 2009;23(4):339–44.
41. Janal MN, Raphael KG, Nayak S, et al. Prevalence of myofascial temporomandibular disorder in US community women. J Oral Rehabil. 2008;35(11):801–9.
42. Schmitter M, Balke Z, Hassel A, et al. The prevalence of myofascial pain and its association with occlusal factors in a threshold country non-patient population. Clin Oral Investig. 2007;11(3):277–81.
43. Obermann M, Katsarava Z. Update on trigeminal neuralgia. Expert Rev Neurother. 2009;9(3):323–9.
44. Manzoni GC, Torelli P. Epidemiology of typical and atypical craniofacial neuralgias. Neurol Sci. 2005;26 Suppl 2:s65–7.
45. Loh HS, Ling SY, Shanmuhasuntharam P, et al. Trigeminal neuralgia A retrospective survey of a sample of patients in Singapore and Malaysia. Aust Dent J. 1998;43(3):188–91.
46. Neto HS, Camilli JA, Marques MJ. Trigeminal neuralgia is caused by maxillary and mandibular nerve entrapment: greater incidence of right-sided facial symptoms is due to the foramen rotundum and foramen ovale being narrower on the right side of the cranium. Med Hypotheses. 2005;65(6):1179–82.
47. Putzki N, Pfriem A, Limmroth V, et al. Prevalence of migraine, tension-type headache and trigeminal neuralgia in multiple sclerosis. Eur J Neurol. 2009;16(2):262–7.
48. Katusic S, Williams DB, Beard CM, et al. Incidence and clinical features of glossopharyngeal neuralgia, Rochester, Minnesota, 1945–1984. Neuroepidemiology. 1991;10(5–6):266–75.
49. Pollock BE, Kondziolka D. Stereotactic radiosurgical treatment of sphenopalatine neuralgia. Case report. J Neurosurg. 1997;87(3):450–3.
50. Ahamed SH, Jones NS. What is Sluder's neuralgia? J Laryngol Otol. 2003;117(6):437–43.
51. Pogrel MA. Summary of: trigeminal nerve injuries in relation to the local anaesthesia in mandibular injections. Br Dent J. 2010;209(9):452–3.
52. Rodríguez-Lozano FJ, Sanchez-Pérez A, Moya-Villaescusa MJ, et al. Neuropathic orofacial pain after dental implant placement: review of the literature and case report. Oral Surg Oral Med Oral Pathol Oral Radiol Endod. 2010;109(4):e8–12.
53. Gialloreti LE, Merito M, Pezzotti P, et al. Epidemiology and economic burden of herpes zoster and post-herpetic neuralgia in Italy: a retrospective, population-based study. BMC Infect Dis. 2010;10:230.
54. Bowsher D. The lifetime occurrence of Herpes zoster and prevalence of post-herpetic neuralgia: a retrospective survey in an elderly population. Eur J Pain. 1999;3(4):335–42.
55. Suzuki N, Mashu S, Toyoda M, et al. Oral burning sensation: prevalence and gender differences in a Japanese population. Pain Pract. 2010;10(4):306–11.
56. Bergdahl M, Bergdahl J. Burning mouth syndrome: prevalence and associated factors. J Oral Pathol Med. 1999;28(8):350–4.
57. Woda A, Pionchon P. A unified concept of idiopathic orofacial pain: pathophysiologic features. J Orofac Pain. 2000;14(3):196–212.
58. Melis M, Lobo SL, Ceneviz C, et al. Atypical odontalgia: a review of the literature. Headache. 2003;43(10):1060–74.
59. Muñoz-Corcuera M, Esparza-Gómez G, González-Moles MA, et al. Oral ulcers: clinical aspects. A tool for dermatologists. Part I. Acute ulcers. Clin Exp Dermatol. 2009;34(4): 289–94.
60. Muñoz-Corcuera M, Esparza-Gómez G, González-Moles MA, et al. Oral ulcers: clinical aspects. A tool for dermatologists. Part II. Chronic ulcers. Clin Exp Dermatol. 2009;34(4): 456–61.
61. Shulman JD, Beach MM, Rivera-Hidalgo F. The prevalence of oral mucosal lesions in US adults: data from the Third National Health and Nutrition Examination Survey, 1988–1994. J Am Dent Assoc. 2004;135(9):1279–86.

62. McCartan BE, Healy CM. The reported prevalence of oral lichen planus: a review and critique. J Oral Pathol Med. 2008;37(8):447–53.
63. Black M, Mignogna MD, Scully C. Number II. Pemphigus vulgaris. Oral Dis. 2005;11(3):119–30.
64. Jurge S, Kuffer R, Scully C, et al. Mucosal disease series. Number VI. Recurrent aphthous stomatitis. Oral Dis. 2006;12(1):1–21.
65. Scully C, Sonis S, Diz PD. Oral mucositis. Oral Dis. 2006;12(3):229–41.
66. Penna PP, Recupero M, Gil C. Influence of psychopathologies on craniomandibular disorders. Braz Dent J. 2009;20(3):226–30.
67. Abetz LM, Savage NW. Burning mouth syndrome and psychological disorders. Aust Dent J. 2009;54(2):84–93. quiz 173.
68. Aggarwal VR, Macfarlane GJ, Farragher TM, et al. Risk factors for onset of chronic oro-facial pain–results of the North Cheshire oro-facial pain prospective population study. Pain. 2010; 149(2):354–9.
69. Rebeiz EE, Rastani K. Sinonasal facial pain. Otolaryngol Clin North Am. 2003; 36(6):1119–26.
70. Chen Y, Dales R, Lin M. The epidemiology of chronic rhinosinusitis in Canadians. Laryngoscope. 2003;113(7):1199–205.
71. Kaliner MA, Osguthorpe JD, Fireman P, et al. Sinusitis: bench to bedside. Current findings, future directions. Otolaryngol Head Neck Surg. 1997;116(6 Pt 2):S1–20.
72. Mohan H, Tahlan A, Mundi I, et al. Non-neoplastic salivary gland lesions: a 15-year study. Eur Arch Otorhinolaryngol. 2010;268(8):1187–90.
73. Dando WE, Branch MA, Maye JP. Headache disability in orofacial pain patients. Headache. 2006;46(2):322–6.
74. Kuncewicz E, Sobieska M, Samborski W. Myofascial pain and tension-type headache. Ann Acad Med Stetin. 2008;54(3):5–9.
75. Teepker M, Schepelmann K. Etiology and diagnostics of headaches and facial pain from the neurological point of view. HNO. 2007;55(7):524–31.
76. Crystal SC, Robbins MS. Epidemiology of tension-type headache. Curr Pain Headache Rep. 2010;14(6):449–54.
77. Yoon MS, Mueller D, Hansen N, et al. Prevalence of facial pain in migraine: a population-based study. Cephalalgia. 2010;30(1):92–6.
78. Davis FG, Kupelian V, Freels S, et al. Prevalence estimates for primary brain tumors in the United States by behavior and major histology groups. Neuro Oncol. 2001;3(3):152–8.
79. Cook RJ, Sharif I, Escudier M. Meningioma as a cause of chronic orofacial pain: case reports. Br J Oral Maxillofac Surg. 2008;46(6):487–9.
80. Bhaya MH, Har-El G. Referred facial pain from intracranial tumors: a diagnostic dilemma. Am J Otolaryngol. 1998;19(6):383–6.
81. Al-Reefy H, Johnson CA, Balfour A, et al. Internal carotid artery aneurysm presenting as sinus pain. J Laryngol Otol. 2007;121(10):1006–8.
82. Trotter MI, Choksey MS. Facial pain with intracranial aneurysm. J R Soc Med. 2000;93(9):479–80. PMID:11089485.
83. Kreiner M, Falace D, Michelis V, et al. Quality difference in craniofacial pain of cardiac vs. dental origin. J Dent Res. 2010;89(9):965–9.
84. Kreiner M, Okeson JP, Michelis V, et al. Craniofacial pain as the sole symptom of cardiac ischemia: a prospective multicenter study. J Am Dent Assoc. 2007;138(1):74–9.
85. Yeh RW, Sidney S, Chandra M, et al. Population trends in the incidence and outcomes of acute myocardial infarction. N Engl J Med. 2010;362(23):2155–65.

Chapter 4
Nociceptive Chemical Mediators in Oral Inflammation

Nalini Vadivelu, Anusha Manje Gowda, Stephen Thorp, Alice Kai, Amarender Vadivelu, and Susan Dabu-Bondoc

Introduction

Orofacial pain is commonly due to inflammation. It is extremely important to understand the chemical mediators of oral inflammation and the pathways of orofacial pain for its effective treatment. This chapter focuses on the pain pathways traversed by impulses causing orofacial pain and the many nociceptive chemical mediators that play a role in oral inflammation.

Nociceptors, the receptors for pain, are unmyelinated nerve endings that are located in bone, skin, muscle, and visceral tissues, the activation of which generates a Ca^{2+} current that depolarizes the distal axonal segment and initiates a self-propagating action potential and an inward current of Na^+. The nociceptors of sensory afferent fibers are activated following tissue injury by the release of prostaglandins mainly the prostaglandin (PGE), which is synthesized by the enzyme cyclooxygenase-2 from the damaged cells, bradykinin from damaged vessels, and cellular mediators including hydrogen and potassium ions. Orthodromic transmission in sensitized afferents initiates the release of peptides like substance P (sP), calcitonin gene-related peptide (CGRP), and cholecystokinin (CCK) within and around

---

N. Vadivelu, M.D. (✉) • S. Thorp, M.D. • S. Dabu-Bondoc, M.D.
Department of Anesthesiology, Yale University School of Medicine and Yale-New Haven Hospital, 333 Cedar Street, 208051, New Haven, CT 06520-8051, USA
e-mail: Nalinivg@gmail.com; Susan.Dabu-Bondoc@yale.edu

A.M. Gowda, M.B.B.S.
Bangalore Medical college and research institute, Bangalore 560003, Karnataka, India

A. Kai, B.A.
Neuroplasticity Unit, National Institutes of Health, Bethesda, MD, USA
e-mail: alicemkai@gmail.com

A. Vadivelu, B.D.S., M.D.S.
Annoor Dental College and Hospital, Muvattupuzha, Kerala 686673, India
e-mail: Amarvadivelu@gmail.com

the site of tissue damage. Substance P further enhances nociceptor excitability through the release of bradykinin, histamine from mast cells, and serotonin (5HT) from platelets. The above factors combine with other mediators such as cytokines and 5HT which results in the inflammatory response and recruits neighboring nociceptors, leading to primary hyperalgesia. Reflex sympathetic efferent responses cause further release of BK and sP which excite nociceptors by the release of noradrenaline, which also results in peripheral vasoconstriction and trophic changes [1].

Pathophysiology of Orofacial Pain

There are three types of primary peripheral afferents: Ab fibers, Ad fibers, and C fibers. Ab fibers are the quickest conducting fibers due to their myelinated quality. Ad fibers are slightly slower, comprising thinner myelinated axons. The slowest conducting fibers are the C fibers consisting of the thinnest and unmyelinated fibers [2].

Trigeminal nerve mostly innervates the orofacial region, and its primary afferent cell bodies are found within the trigeminal ganglion which consists mostly of Ad fibers and C fibers [3]. The Ab fibers of the trigeminal region respond to pressure and light touch, while pain acts as a stimulus to the less conducting Ad fibers and C fibers, which are jointly termed nociceptors, the excitation of which causes considerable release of sP, which activates neurokinin-1 receptors and thereby modulates sensitivity to pain [4]. These nociceptors can be further classified into mechano-nociceptors, thermo-nociceptors, and chemo-nociceptors. Thermo-nociceptors contain vanilloid receptor 1-like receptors that contribute to the pain due to extreme temperatures [5]. Mechano-nociceptors, which are sensitive to mechanical stimuli, are located in the root pulp and are lined with epithelial Na^+ channels that contribute to sharp pain produced by liquid motion in the dentinal tubules [6]. Chemo-nociceptors are sensitive to chemicals.

The modulation of these nociceptors is either mechanical or chemical. Canine studies have shown that the threshold for mechano-nociception can increase sensitization because it may be lowered by periodontal inflammation [7]. It is possible that this is due to the hydrodynamic mechanism (which activates the nociceptors by increasing pressure on the pulp [8]) of inflammation in the noncompliant environment in the dentine-encased pulp. In addition, there is substantial peripheral and central modulation due to the various neuropeptides released following tissue damage, and it is localized within the trigeminal ganglia. Peptides such as sP and calcitonin-related peptide are crucial in sensitizing the nociceptors: this leads to allodynia, the pain to innocuous stimuli, and hyperalgesia, increased sensitivity to painful stimuli [9].

The primary afferent neurons terminate in the trigeminal spinal tract nucleus in the brain stem. The trigeminal spinal tract nucleus is made up of three subnuclei: the subnucleus oralis, subnucleus interpolaris, and subnucleus caudalis. The subnucleus caudalis is structurally comparable to the spinal dorsal horn and hence often called the trigeminal dorsal horn [10]. This subnucleus functions as the main brain stem relay and is a critical central structure for the modulation of nociception.

The subnucleus oralis and subnucleus interpolaris both receive a versatile input from all three types of fibers, particularly from the quickly conducting Ab fibers. The central neurons found within these subnuclei are further subdivided into nociceptive specific neurons. This consists of either Ad fibers and C fibers that respond only to noxious stimuli or all the three fiber types that respond to both noxious and innocuous stimuli [11]. Deep pain is attributed to the convergence of various types of receptors into a central nociceptive neuron. The intricacy of this convergence results in the misreading of the original sensation, leading to allodynia or hyperalgesia [12]. In addition, various other studies have also found that the transition zone between the subnuclei caudalis and the subnuclei interpolaris also contributes to the central processing of deep orofacial nociception [13].

From the brain stem, the orofacial impulses are conducted through the thalamus to the cortex. In the thalamus, mainly the posterior nucleus, ventral posterior nucleus, and intralaminar nucleus, nociceptive specific neurons and wide dynamic range neurons are located. The ventral posterior nucleus is involved in localization of pain to a region, and the intralaminar nucleus is responsible for the affective and motivational dimension to pain and identification of stimuli as pain is caused by the posterior nucleus. In effect, the lateral thalamus projects to the somatosensory cerebral cortex to narrow down and identify the location of the pain, and the medial thalamus projects to neighboring areas such as the hypothalamus and the cingulated gyrus in order to associate the pain with their relevant emotions [14].

Transduction, Conduction, and Transmission of Nociceptors

Transduction

The activity of nociceptors can be classified into that of transduction, conduction, and transmission. Transduction [15] is the response of peripheral nociceptors to noxious impulses caused by traumatic, mechanical, chemical, or thermal stimuli that are converted within the distal nociceptors into a depolarization current mediated by Ca^2. Cellular damage and neurohormonal response to the injury in the skin, fascia, bone, muscle, and ligaments cause the release of intracellular H^+ and K^+ ions, in addition to arachidonic acid (AA) from cell membranes that have been lysed and other noxious mediators. The accumulated AA activates and up regulates the cyclooxygenase-2 enzyme isoform (COX-2), which leads to conversion of AA into biologically active metabolites like prostaglandin E2 (PGE2) and prostaglandin G2 (PGG2), followed by prostaglandin H2 (PGH2). These metabolites and the intracellular H^+ and K^+ ions cause the sensitization of peripheral nociceptors that initiates inflammatory responses leading to pain and an increase in the swelling of the tissue at the site of injury [16].

Other important primary and secondary noxious sensitizers that are released following tissue injury are 5-hydroxytryptamine (5-HT) [17], bradykinin (BK) [18], and histamine [19]. The 5-HT released in response to thermal stimuli activates peripheral 5-HT2a receptors causing sensitization of primary afferent neurons leading to mechanical allodynia and thermal hyperalgesia [20]. G-protein-coupled receptors [21] B1 and B2, which are located in the primary nociceptors, mediate bradykinin's role in peripheral sensitization. The receptor–G-protein complex, when activated by BK and kallidin, leads to increase of nociceptor excitability by causing inward Na^+ flux and reduced outward K^+ currents. The resulting primary hyperalgesia is due to the increase in nociceptor irritability, increase in vascular permeability, initiation of neurogenic edema, and activation of adjacent nociceptor endings caused by these locally released substances. In addition, bradykinin, 5-HT, and other primary mediators excite orthodromic transmission in sensitized nerve endings and initiate the release of various peptides and neurokinins like CGRP [22], sP [23], and CCK [24] in and around the injury site.

Substance P enhances sensitization of peripheral nociceptors by inducing further release of histamine from mast cells, bradykinin, and 5-HT through a feedback loop mechanism. Calcitonin gene-related protein, a 37 amino acid peptide, is present in the central and peripheral terminals of greater than 35 % of Ad fibers and 50 % of C fibers [25]. Similar to sP, CGRP [26] produced in the cell bodies of primary nociceptors found in the dorsal root ganglion initiates mechanical and thermal hyperalgesia. CGRP released at peripheral endings has several effects including the inhibition of its peripheral metabolic breakdown, which prolongs the effect of sP [27] and histamine-induced vasodilation and inflammatory extravasation.

Acute tissue injury leads to an increase in the production and release of proinflammatory cytokines including IL-1b and IL-6, which play a critical role in intensifying the edema and irritation associated with pain caused by inflammation [28]. Inflammatory mediators and these proinflammatory cytokines activate transducer molecules including the transient receptor potential (TRP) ion channels [21]. Up to eight types of TRP ion channels have been discovered, and the response of each varies depending on mediators activated by the thermal, chemical, or traumatic stimuli within the surrounding microenvironment. The 4-unit TRP-VI/capsaicin ion channel receptor consists of a central ion channel that allows inward flow of Na^+ and Ca^{2+} after being activated by H^+ ions, heat, and presence of capsaicin [29]. This inward ion flux of Ca^+ activates the generator potential [19], which causes summation and depolarization of distal axonal component. The resulting action potential is conducted centrally to the dorsal horn axon terminals.

Conduction

Conduction is the propagation of action potentials through myelinated and unmyelinated nerve fibers, from peripheral nociceptive endings. Nociceptive and nonnoxious nerve fibers can be classified by the extent of myelination, diameter, and conduction velocity. Ab fibers are the nonnoxious special sensory fibers of greatest diameter that are found in somatic structures like skin and joints. The nociceptive fibers are of two varieties—the Ad fibers and C fibers, which are distributed in skin and other tissues. The Ad fibers propagate the "first pain," which is defined as a sharp, localized stinging sensation of a duration up to 1 s. This "first pain" serves to warn the person of potential injury and causes withdrawal response. The C fibers, also known as high-threshold polymodal nociceptive fibers, are activated by mechanical, thermal, and chemical stimuli and are responsible for the perception of "second pain" that has a prolonged latency lasting from seconds to minutes [30]. It is described as a non-localized stabbing, burning sensation that becomes progressively more comfortable. Ion channels that are located in nociceptive axons and their terminal endings seem to have particular roles in conduction of noxious impulses. Axonal Na^+ ion channels are classified as either sensitive or resistant (TTX-r) to biotoxin tetrodotoxin of the puffer fish. Axonal conduction in nociceptive fibers results in secretion of excitatory amino acids (EAAs) and peptide neurotransmitters from presynaptic terminals in the dorsal horn. The release of EAAs in these nerve terminals is brought about by neuronal-type (N-type) calcium channels, which are voltage-gated channels composed of four subunits that open following depolarization allowing the rapid influx of Ca^{2+} ions. These channels can be blocked by conotoxins including ziconotide.

Transmission

Transmission is defined as the transfer of noxious impulses from primary nociceptors to cells located in the dorsal horn of spinal cord. Ad and C fibers are axons of the unipolar neurons that have nociceptive endings which enter the dorsal horn and branch within Lissauer's tract and ultimately synapse with second-order cells that are situated mostly in Rexed's laminae II known as substantia gelatinosa and V known as nucleus proprius. There are two kinds of second-order dorsal horn neurons, consisting of the nociceptive specific (NS) neurons and WDR. Nociceptive specific neurons found in lamina I are stimulated only by noxious impulses from C fibers, while WDR that are mostly found in lamina I are responsive to both noxious and innocuous stimuli. There is a wide range of responses that are dependent on frequency stimulation: low-frequency stimulation of C fibers leads to sensory transmission not related to pain, while high-frequency stimulation of WDR neurons results in progressive increases in discharge and transmission of painful impulses [31].

The rapid transmission through synapses and accelerated neuronal depolarization is due to excitatory amino acids like glutamate (Glu) and aspartate. Excitatory amino acids stimulate ionotropic amino-3-hydroxy-5-methyl-4-propionic acid (AMPA) and kainite (Kar) receptors, which modulate the influx of K^+ and Na^+ ions along with intraneural voltage potential. These receptors are rather impervious to other cations like Ca^{2+}. Each AMPA receptor contains the central cation channel surrounded by four subunits that have intrinsic binding sites for glutamate. The interaction of agonists with two or more binding sites on the receptor results in activation and opening of the channel, permitting Na⁺ influx into the cell [32], leading to rapid transmission of noxious impulses to supraspinal sites of perception. Kainate receptors also regulate the influx of Na⁺ and K⁺ ions and are responsible for postsynaptic excitation. However, KAR receptors also seem to be involved in transmission of synaptic signals that follows brief noxious excitation. In addition, KAR receptors may increase the efficacy of synaptic transmission by multiplying the likelihood of discharge from second-order neurons in conditions of ongoing excitation.

Under conditions of high-frequency noxious stimulation, AMPA and KAR receptors activate the priming of N-methyl-D-aspartic acid (NMDA) receptors that is voltage mediated [33, 34]. The NMDA receptor is a ligand-specific ion channel that is voltage gated. It consists of four subunits—two NR2 units with sites for glutamate binding on its extracellular portions and two NRI units with binding sites for glycine and an allosteric site that is reactive to zinc ions. The receptor regulates the influx of Na⁺ and Ca²⁺ ions and the outflow of K⁺ ions through its intrinsic ion channel. Each subunit has a considerable cytoplasmic part that can be altered by protein kinases and an outer allosteric component that is modifiable by zinc ions. Activation of these receptors requires an AMPA-induced membrane depolarization with a positive change in intracellular voltage in addition to the binding of aspartate or glutamate to the receptor. AMPA receptors that are activated result in excitatory postsynaptic potentials (EPSPs) that span for several hundred milliseconds [35] and accumulate to produce a depolarization that removes a Mg²⁺ "plug" that inhibits the NMDA ion channel, permitting Ca²⁺ ion influx. The accumulation of Ca²⁺ ions leads to series of neurochemical and neurophysiological events that influence processing of acute pain. In a process known as "windup" that specially involves excitation of dorsal horn neurons independent of transcription, second-order spinal neurons become highly sensitized and fire rapidly without the need for further activation.

Studies by Woolf have found that the activation of NMDA receptors, the process of "windup," and central sensitization play a critical role in clinical hyperalgesia and can be incited by trauma, nerve injury, and inflammation. The central sensitization is found in supraspinal regions of the CAN that include the amygdala, anterior cingulated gyrus, and rostroventral medulla [36]. The influx of Ca²⁺ ions also activates inducible enzymes that include COX-2 and nitric oxide synthase (NOS). Peptides including sP and CGRP result in the delayed and prolonged depolarization of second-order dorsal horn neurons. When sP binds to metabotropic neurokinin 1 (NK-1), NMDARs are activated: this seems essential for the establishment of long-term potentiation (LTP) [37]. Upon stimulation of NK-1, phosphokinase A (PKA) and cyclic adenosine monophosphate (cAMP) are synthesized which mediate various changes in the cell such as the slow priming of NMDA receptors, genome activation, and second-messenger cascades. The increase in intracellular and extracellular PGE and NO and the synthesis of acute-phase proteins lead to transcription-dependent central sensitization and are associated with responses that facilitate changes in neural plasticity.

Conclusion

To prevent neural plasticity and long-term orofacial pain it is therefore important to control inflammation and resultant morbidity at the earliest. The effects of neurotransmitters can be blocked at specific levels in the pain pathways of the head, neck, and face region that are involved in the development of orofacial pain by medical and interventional pain management. Controlling inflammation and blocking of the pain pathways can result in decrease of peripheral and central sensitization and LTP of pain.

Acknowledgement The authors wish to thank Nirmal Kumar, Amarender Vadivelu, Gopal Kodumudi, and Vijay Kodumudi for their help in the preparation of the manuscript.

Conflict of Interest None declared.

References

1. Vadivelu N, Whitney CJ, Sinatra RS. Pain pathways and acute pain processing. New York: Cambridge Univ. Press; 2009.
2. Hunt CC. Relation of function to diameter in afferent fibers of muscle nerves. J Gen Physiol. 1954;38(1):117–31.
3. Dubner R, Sessle BJ, Store AT. The neural basis of oral and facial function. New York: Plenum; 1978.
4. Jessel TM. Substance P, in nociceptive sensory neurons. Ciba Found Symp. 1982;91:225–48. Review.
5. Ichikawa H, Sugimoto T. Vanilloid receptor 1-like receptor-immunoreactive primary sensory neurons in the rat trigeminal nervous system. Neuroscience. 2000;101(3):719–25.
6. Ichikawa H, Fukuda T, Terayama R, Yamaai T, Kuboki T, Sugimoto T. Immunohistochemical localization of gamma and beta subunits of epithelial Na+ channel in the rat molar tooth pulp. Brain Res. 2005;1065(1–2):138–41. Epub 2005 Nov 17.
7. Matsumoto H. Effects of pulpal inflammation on the activities of periodontal mechanoreceptive afferent fibers. Kokubyo Gakkai Zasshi. 2010;77(2):115–20.
8. Mathews B, Sessle BJ. Peripheral mechanisms of orofacial pain. In: Sessle BK, Lavigne GL, Lund JP, et al., editors. Orofacial pain. 2nd ed. Chicago: Quintessence; 2008. p. 27–43.
9. Meyer RA, Ringkamp M, Campbell JN, et al. Peripheral mechanisms of cutaneous nociception. In: McMahon SB, Koltzenburg M, editors. Wall and Melzacks textbook of pain. 5th ed. Amsterdam: Elsevier; 2006. p. 3–34.
10. Gobel S, Bennett GJ, Allen B, Humphrey E, Seltzer Z, Abdelmoumene M, Hayashi H, Hoffert MJ. Synaptic connectivity of substantia gelatinosa neurons with reference to potential termination site of descending axons. In: Sjolund B, Bjorkland A, editors. Brain stem control of spinal mechanisms. NewYork: Elsevier/North Holland; 1982.
11. Tenebaum HC, Mock D, Gordon AS, Goldberg MB, Grossi ML, Locker D, Davis KD. Sensory and affective components of orofacial pain: is it all in your brain? Crit Rev Oral Biol Med. 2001;12(6):455–68. Review.
12. Ness TJ, Gebhart GF. Visceral pain: a review of experimental studies. Pain. 1990;41(2):167–234. Review; PMID: 2195438.

13. Shimizu K, Guo W, Wang H, Zou S, LaGraize SC, Iwata K, Wei F, Dubner R, Ren K. Differential involvement of trigeminal transition zone and laminated subnucleus caudalis in orofacial deep and cutaneous hyperalgesia: the effects of interleukin-10 and glial inhibitors. Mol Pain. 2009;5:75. PubMed PMID: 20025765; PubMed Central PMCID: PMC2806354.
14. Willis WD. Nociceptive functions of thalamic neurons. In: Sterlade M, Jones EG, McCormick DA, editors. Thalamus. Oxford: Elsevier Science; 1997.
15. Ji RR, Woolf CJ. Neuronal plasticity and signal transduction in nociceptive neurons: implications for the initiation and maintenance of pathological pain. Neurobiol Dis. 2001;8(1):1–10.
16. Ito S, Okuda-Ashitaka E, Minami T. Central and peripheral roles of prostaglandins in pain and their interactions with novel neuropeptides nociceptin and nocistatin. Neurosci Res. 2001;41(4):299–332.
17. Funk CD. Prostaglandins and leukotrienes: advances in eicosanoid biology. Science. 2001;294(5584):1871–5.
18. Millan MJ. Serotonin and pain: evidence that activation of 5-HT1A receptors does not elicit antinociception against noxious thermal, mechanical and chemical stimuli in mice. Pain. 1994;58(1):45–61.
19. Wang H, Kohno T, Amaya F, Brenner GJ, Ito N, Allchorne A, et al. Bradykinin produces pain hypersensitivity by potentiating spinal cord glutamatergic synaptic transmission. J Neurosci. 2005;25(35):7986–92.
20. Sasaki M, Obata H, Kawahara K, Saito S, Goto F. Peripheral 5-HT2A receptor antagonism attenuates primary thermal hyperalgesia and secondary mechanical allodynia after thermal injury in rats. Pain. 2006;122(1–2):130–6.
21. Woolf CJ, Salter MW. Neuronal plasticity: increasing the gain in pain. New York, NY: Science; 2000. p. 1765–9.
22. Bennett AD, Chastain KM, Hulsebosch CE. Alleviation of mechanical and thermal allodynia by CGRP(8-37) in a rodent model of chronic central pain. Pain. 2000;86(1–2):163–75.
23. Liu H, Mantyh PW, Basbaum AI. NMDA-receptor regulation of substance P release from primary afferent nociceptors. Nature. 1997;386(6626):721–4.
24. Noble F, Derrien M, Roques BP. Modulation of opioid antinociception by CCK at the supraspinal level: evidence of regulatory mechanisms between CCK and enkephalin systems in the control of pain. Br J Pharmacol. 1993;109(4):1064–70.
25. McCarthy PW, Lawson SN. Cell type and conduction velocity of rat primary sensory neurons with calcitonin gene-related peptide-like immunoreactivity. Neuroscience. 1990;34(3):623–32.
26. Evans BN, Rosenblatt MI, Mnayer LO, Oliver KR, Dickerson IM. CGRP-RCP, a novel protein required for signal transduction at calcitonin gene-related peptide and adrenomedullin receptors. J Biol Chem. 2000;275(40):31438–43.
27. Tzabazis AZ, Pirc G, Votta-Velis E, Wilson SP, Laurito CE, Yeomans DC. Antihyperalgesic effect of a recombinant herpes virus encoding antisense for calcitonin gene-related peptide. Anesthesiology. 2007;106(6):1196–203.
28. Bessler H, Shavit Y, Mayburd E, Smirnov G, Beilin B. Postoperative pain, morphine consumption, and genetic polymorphism of Il-1beta and Il-1 receptor antagonist. Neurosci Lett. 2006;404(1–2):154–8.
29. Winter J, Bevan S, Campbell EA. Capsaicin and pain mechanisms. Br J Anaesth. 1995;75(2):157–68.
30. Djouhri L, Koutsikou S, Fang X, McMullan S, Lawson SN. Spontaneous pain, both neuropathic and inflammatory, is related to frequency of spontaneous firing in intact C-fiber nociceptors. J Neurosci. 2006;26(4):1281–92.
31. Hogan QH, Abram SE. Neural blockade for diagnosis and prognosis: a review. Anesthesiology. 1997;86(1):216–41.
32. Malinow R, Malenka RC. AMPA receptor trafficking and synaptic plasticity. Annu Rev Neurosci. 2002;25:103–26.
33. Woolf CJ. An overview of the mechanisms of hyperalgesia. Pulm Pharmacol. 1995;8(4–5):161–7.

34. Mannion RJ, Woolf CJ. Pain mechanisms and management: a central perspective. Clin J Pain. 2000;16(3 Suppl):S144–56.
35. Silvilotti LG, Thompson SW, Woolf CJ. Rate of rise of the cumulative depolarization evoked by repetitive stimulation of small-caliber afferents is a predictor of action potential windup in rat spinal neurons in vitro. J Neurophysiol. 1993;69(5):1621–31.
36. Porreca F, Ossipov MH, Gebhart GF. Chronic pain and medullary descending facilitation. Trends Neurosci. 2002;25(6):319–25.
37. Ikeda H, Heinke B, Ruscheweyh R, Sandkuhler J. Synaptic plasticity in spinal lamina I projection neurons that mediate hyperalgesia. Science. 2003;299(5610):1237–40.

Chapter 5
Dental Sleep Medicine and the Use of Oral Devices

Ghabi A. Kaspo

Introduction

Approximately, one-third of life is spent sleeping. Sleep is very important to humans; disruption and/or deprivation of sleep typically results in adverse physiological effects. The overall prevalence of sleep problems may be as high as 30 % in children and adults and even higher in elderly people. Obstructive sleep apnea (OSA) is associated with higher risks for HT, coronary heart disease, stroke, congestive heart failure, atrial fibrillation, impotence, mortality, and behavior and cognitive problems [1]. Sleep apnea [2] leading to excessive daytime hypersomnolence may be responsible for many job-related injuries, and it is estimated that people with sleep apnea are ten times more likely to die in a car accident than someone without sleep apnea.

It is also known that adequate sleep is needed to maintain alertness, heal the body, and assist with memory and learning. The physiologic and neurochemical activities of the sleep and awake states need to be better understood. However, the complexity and study of sleep require a comprehensive understanding of the physiology, neuroanatomy, neurochemistry, and associated mechanisms by which these areas interact.

The social and economic impact of sleep disorders is estimated at $16 billion annually for health care expenses and $50 billion annually regarding lost productivity. Sleep disorders are considered one of the most common health problems, and yet it has been demonstrated that between 82 and 98 % of adults with sleep-related breathing disorders (SRBD) are undiagnosed.

G.A. Kaspo, D.D.S., D.Orth. (✉)
Clinical instructor of the St. Joseph Hospital-Oakland Dental Residency Program,
Staff at St. Joseph Mercy Hospital of Pontiac and Wayne State University,
3144 John R Road, Suite 100, Troy, MI 48083, USA

Wayne State University - Detroit Medical Centers, 31000 Telegraph Road, Suite 110,
Bingham Farms, MI 48025, USA
e-mail: gakaspodds@gmail.com

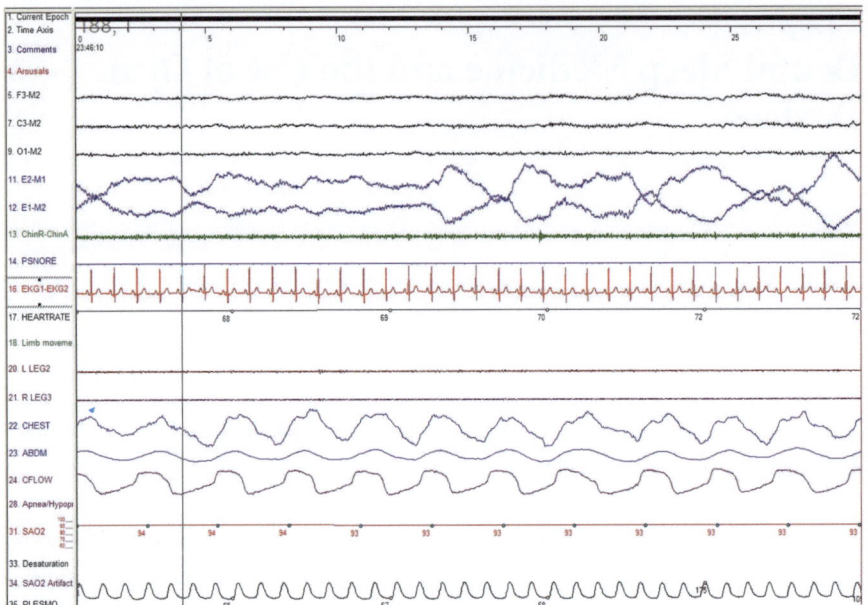

Fig. 5.1 Stage (N1) (courtesy of George Zureikat, MD)

Sleep disturbances can be classified into one of the four groups: insomnia, hypersomnia, parasomnia, and sleep–wake schedule disorders. Insomnia [3] describes a condition in which a patient is tired and desires to sleep, yet suffers from a combination of difficulties involving falling asleep, maintaining sleep, and awakening too early. Hypersomnia, on the other hand, describes a condition in which a patient remains sleepy, usually despite adequate sleep time. Parasomnias are described events occurring during sleep, and sleep–wake schedule disorders (known also as circadian rhythm abnormalities) reflect a situation in which a patient sleeps at undesired times.

Sleep Architect

The discovery of electroencephalography in 1928 by Berger provided a quantum leap for sleep research. In applying the new methods to measure EEG activities in sleeping people, or animals, it was revealed that the transition from wakefulness [4] to sleep is accompanied by specific and well-characterized changes in brain wave activities (Fig. 5.1). EEG has allowed widespread investigations of the brain mechanism controlling sleep and wakefulness [5] by several investigators [4–6].

During sleep, there are periods of physiological and autonomic activation reaching waking levels. EEG and other physiological recordings during sleep define two distinct states of sleep: the time of rapid eye movement (REM) [7] and that of non-REM

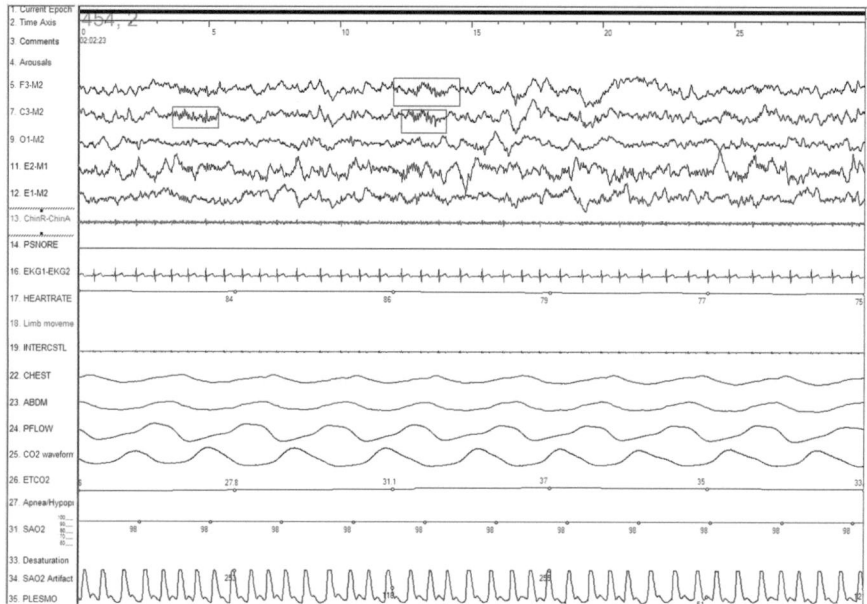

Fig. 5.2 Stage (N2) spindles (courtesy of George Zureikat, MD)

(NREM). The second is divided into four stages: stage (N1) also called light sleep, stage (N2) also called consolidated sleep, and stages (N3) and (N4) also called deep or slow-wave sleep. Division of sleep into these stages relies on electroencephalogram (EEG), electromyography (EMG), and electrooculography (EOG).

The different EEG patterns that are characteristic of NREM sleep stages are shown in Figs. 5.1, 5.2, 5.3, and 5.4. Stage (N1) is characterized by relatively low-amplitude alpha waves and activity intermixed with episodes of alpha activity. In stage (N2) there are K-complex wave forms and sleep spindles, whereas stages (N3) and (N4) are dominated by an increased amount of slow waves and high amplitude of delta activity.

NREM: Historically, this sleep pattern is divided into four distinct stages on the bases of characteristic of brain waves and physiologic activities.

Stage (N1): This stage reflects a change in brain wave activity from rhythmic alpha waves to mixed-frequency waves as the individual passes from wakefulness to the initiation of sleep. Stage (N1) comprises about 2–5 % of the total sleep time, and it is considered to be a drowsy or a light sleep stage from which one can usually be awakened easily. Sudden muscle contractions can occur in this stage, and the individual may also experience a sensation of falling.

Stage (N2): Although this begins to be a deeper stage of sleep with a reduction of heart rate and body temperature, it is still regarded as being light with mixed-frequency EEG activity. He or she can again be easily aroused or awakened, although an additional amount of stimulus is needed as compared to stage (N1). This stage

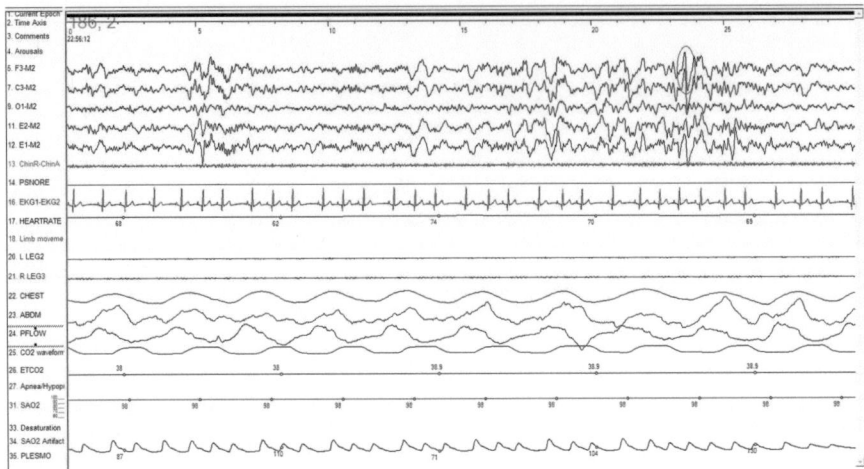

Fig. 5.3 Stage N2 K-complex (courtesy of George Zureikat, MD)

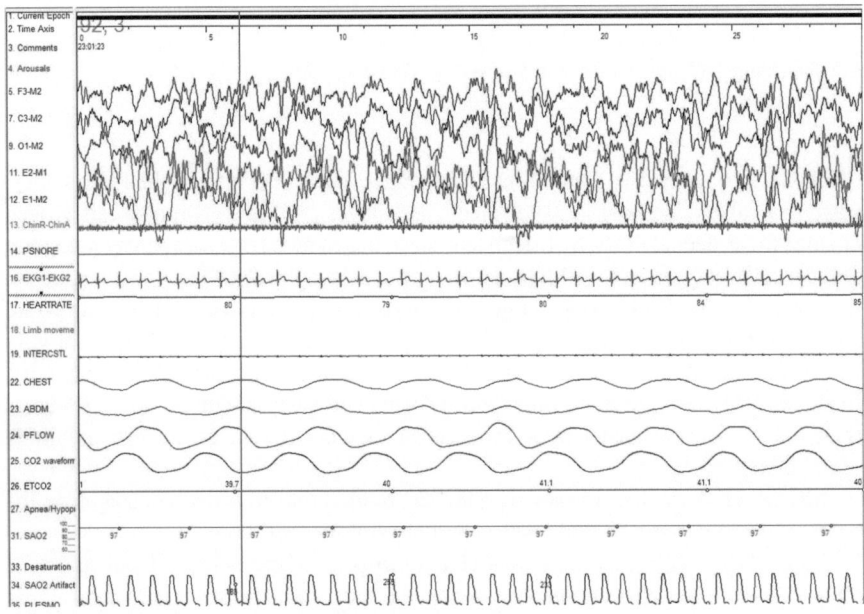

Fig. 5.4 Stage (N3) (courtesy of George Zureikat, MD)

comprises about 45–55 % of the total sleep time. Unique and significant features in the EEG activity of this stage are the presence of K-complex wave forms and sleep spindles, the latter of which have been postulated as being associated with memory consolidation. The K-complex may appear as a result of some type of stimulation, such as noise, or it may appear spontaneously.

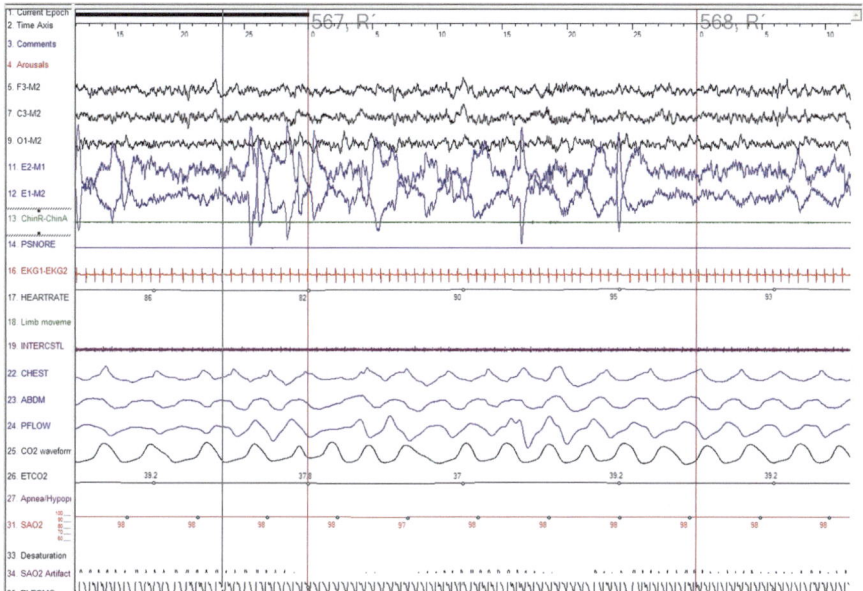

Fig. 5.5 Stage R (courtesy of George Zureikat, MD)

Stages (N3) and (N4): These two NREM stages have their own unique brain wave forms, but they are usually viewed as one stage of sleep, being referred to as slow-wave sleep, deep sleep, or restorative sleep. Because of their unique EEG wave forms, they are also known as delta sleep. Together, they comprise about 13–23 % of the total sleep time. Stage (N4) reflects the highest threshold for awakening from sleep relative to the other NREM stages.

REM Sleep

REM sleep is also referred to as dream sleep. Although it comprises only about 20–25 % of the total sleep time, this state recurs several times throughout the overall cyclical activity of NREM and REM states during a sleep period. In normal sleep, each subsequent recurring REM period is longer than the prior REM period.

EEG activity is increased with a characteristic "sawtooth" wave form and can also appear similar to wakefulness relative to mixed frequency (Fig. 5.5). There is a concomitant increase in heart rate, respiration, blood pressure, and jerky eye movements. During this state of increased cerebral activity, there may be a near immobility or paralysis of the muscles in the limbs, which has been thought to be a preventive mechanism of the individual to not physically act out his or her dreams during sleep. REM sleep may also be contributory to memory consolidation.

Table 5.1 New sleep scoring table	Stage W (wakefulness)
	Stage N1 (NREM1)
	Stage N2 (NREM2)
	Stage N3 (NREM3; this replaces NREM stages 3 and 4)
	Stage R (REM)

REM sleep may be further regarded as two phases: tonic and phasic. However, a typical sleep study report will not make a distinction between these two phases.

Tonic REM is a unique phase by virtue of the following characteristics: hypotonia (partial loss of muscle tone) of the skeletal muscles that approaches near paralysis and desynchronized EEG activity with widespread neural activation or wake-like EEG activity.

Phasic REM is also unique because it occurs sporadically instead of continuously, and it reflects the following characteristics: bursts of REMs in all directions, transient swings in blood pressure and heart rate along with tongue movement and irregular respiration, myoclonus (muscular jerks), twitching of the chin, and limb movements.

Alternative Sleep Scoring/Staging

In 2007, a new method of scoring sleep studies led to a revision in sleep staging; the new scoring is explained in the new sleep scoring table (Table 5.1) comparing to the old score in parenthesis.

Cycles and Hours of Sleep

Sleep patterns and architecture change for individuals throughout life. From infancy to old age, these changes are dynamic and distinct, relative to sleep initiation and maintenance and the amount of time for each sleep stage.

During normal sleep, man typically cycles through the NREM and REM sleep stages four to six times per sleep period. In children, these stages are shorter and occur at about 50–60-min intervals. In the adult, regardless of the age, these stages occur at about 90-min intervals. In addition, children have different proportions of REM and NREM sleep as well as different numbers of hours of sleep. A newborn typically sleeps 16–18 h, and 50 % of this sleep time is REM sleep. Slow-wave sleep (NREM stages 3 and 4) is at its maximum in young children since this is when growth hormone is secreted.

With age, slow-wave sleep decreases, which appears to begin after adolescence. After the age of 70, slow-wave sleep is minimal or, in some cases, nonexistent. In addition, the elderly spend more time in bed and less time actively sleeping [8].

Also as people age, they often begin to adjust the time that they go to bed to an earlier and earlier hour. The result is that they have an increased potential to wake up earlier in the morning, which is a condition termed advanced sleep phase syndrome. In this syndrome, the individual purposely adjusts the sleep–wake schedule by attempting to initiate sleep in advance of the circadian rhythm. As such, the intentional adjustment is not synchronized with this internal biological rhythm.

With the aging process, the typical sleep architecture becomes more fragmented with increased awakenings or arousals during the sleep period and people tend to subsequently have an increased risk for sleep disorders, including SRBD and insomnia. With SRBD, the musculature that supports the airway becomes more relaxed during sleep, and this lends itself to increased collapsibility. Therefore, as one's age increases, the potential risk for SRBD is increased. The role of the dentist is significant for the recognition of OSA and for the management of this sleep disorder with oral appliance (OA) therapy.

Sleep–Wake Cycle

Circadian Rhythm

Humans tend to alternate between a period of wakefulness [9] lasting approximately 16 h and a continuous block of 8 h of sleep. Most mammals sleep around a 24-h cycle that is driven by clock genes that control the circadian rhythm [10] (known as process C). Light helps humans synchronize their rhythm with the cycles of the sun and moon by sending a retinal signal (melanopsin) to the hypothalamic suprachiasmatic nucleus. The suprachiasmatic nucleus that acts as a pacemaker to control the circadian timing function [11].

The investigation of process C uses biologic markers to assess a given individual's rhythm. A slight drop (hundredths of a degree centigrade) in body temperature and a rise in salivary and blood melatonin and growth hormone release peaking around midnight in the 24-h cycle are key indications of the acrophase (high peak) of process C. Interestingly, corticotropins (adrenocorticotropic hormone and cortisol) reach a nadir (lowest level) during the first hour of sleep. They then reach an acrophase in the second half of the sleep cycle process C that can also be studied using temperature recordings in relation to hormone release and polygraphy to measure brain, muscle, and heart activities.

Ultradian Rhythm

Under the 24-h process C of sleep and wakefulness, sleep onset and maintenance are governed by an ultradian cycle of three to five periods in which the brain, muscles, and autonomic cardiac and respiratory activities fluctuate. These cycles consist of REM, sleep (active stage), and NREM sleep (light and deep stages). The REM stage is known as paradoxical sleep in Europe.

In humans, a clear decline in electrical brain and muscle activities as well as heart rhythm is observed from wakefulness to sleep onset. This decline is associated with a synchronization of brain waves toward stage I of sleep. Stage I is a transitional period between wakefulness and sleep. Stage 2 sleep then begins, accounting for about 50–60 % of total sleep duration. Stage 2 sleep is characterized by two EEG signals, K-complexes (brief, high-amplitude brain waves) and spindles (rapid, springlike EEG waves), both of which are described as sleep-promoting and sleep-preserving factors. Sleep stages I and 2 are categorized as light sleep.

Next, sleep enters a quiet period known as deep sleep or stages 3 and 4. These stages are characterized by slow, high-amplitude brain wave activities. Stages 3 and 4 are usually scored together and are characterized by a dominance of slow-wave activity (delta sleep=0.5–4.5 Hz). This sleep period is associated with the so-called sleep recovery process.

Finally, sleep enters an ascension period and rapidly turns into either light sleep or REM sleep. REM sleep is associated with a reduction in the tone of postural muscles (which is poorly described as "atonia" in literature but is in fact hypotonia because muscle tone is never zero) and a rise in heart rate and brain activity to levels that frequently surpass the rates observed during wakefulness. Humans can dream in all stages of sleep, but REM dreams may involve intensely vivid imagery with fantastic and creative content. During REM sleep, the body is typically in a paralyzed-like state (muscle hypotonia). Otherwise, dreams with intense emotional content and motor activity might cause body movements that could injure individuals and their sleep partners.

An understanding of the presence of ultradian sleep cycles is relevant because certain pathologic events occur during sleep, including the following sleep disorders:

Most periodic body movements (leg or arm) and jaw movements, such as sleep bruxism, are observed in stage 2 sleep and with less frequency in REM sleep.

Sleep-related breathing events, such as apnea and hypopnea (cessation or reduction of breathing), are observed in stage 2 and REM sleep. Acted dreams with risk of body injury, diagnosed as the sleep movement disorder and REM behavior disorder, occur during REM sleep.

Sleep Disorders and Their Assessment

The second edition of the International Classification of Sleep Disorders (ICSD) lists 85 sleep disorders in eight major categories:

- Insomnias
- Sleep-related breathing disorders
- Hypersomnia

- Circadian rhythm disorders
- Parasomnias
- Sleep-related movement disorders
- Isolated symptoms as a category
- Other sleep disorders

Insomnias

Insomnia is defined by a difficulty in sleep initiation, duration, consolidation, or quality that occurs despite adequate time and opportunity for sleep and results in some form of daytime impairment.

Insomnia is the most commonly reported sleep disorder. It is subjectively reported by the patient and can typically include difficulty getting to sleep, awakening from sleep earlier than the desired wake-up time, and then getting back to sleep as well as the feeling of a poor quality of sleep. These subjective complaints are reported even though the individual has had ample time for sleep, and the end result is typically excessive daytime sleepness (EDS) or fatigue along with its subsequent adverse impact on daytime function and quality of wakefulness[7]. These subjective complaints may be generally confirmed through the objective findings of a polysomnography (PSG) sleep study, but PSG is not the standard of care for the definitive diagnosis of insomnia.

Although the etiology of insomnia is not completely understood, it appears to involve biological, psychological, and social elements, and it can be regarded as a condition of hyperarousal.

Sleep-Related Breathing Disorders

Abnormal breathing during sleep is increasingly recognized as a clinical problem. Patients with lung disease, such as asthma and chronic obstructive pulmonary disease (COPD), may develop periods of even worse oxygen desaturations of the body's tissues during sleep. However, decreased frequency and depth of breathing during sleep-related breathing disorder are mostly applied to sleep apnea and hypopnea syndrome.

Snoring

Snoring is an acoustic phenomenon. Usually it happens on inhalation and is caused by fluttering and vibration of the soft tissues of the upper airway; the snoring described here occurs without episodes of apnea or hypoventilation.

Snoring is very common with an occurrence in 24 % of adult females and 40 % of adult males. Because snoring is usually more of a complaint for the bed partner than it is for the snorer, the noise is typically the primary reason for seeking a medical consultation. Not all individuals who snore have OSA, but those individuals with OSA generally demonstrate a snoring component during their sleep period. Thus, it is possible for snoring to be a precursor to OSA.

When snoring occurs without any sleep pattern fragmentation or respiratory apneic or hypopneic episodes, it is often referred to as primary (benign) snoring. Whereas individuals with OSA will report the classic descriptions of EDS or insomnia, individuals with primary or benign snoring will not have these experiences. However, snoring may also be associated with many of the same symptoms as OSA.

Unfortunately, the individual who snores may not be aware of the association of OSA symptoms and snoring, and thus some snorers may also experience EDS along with associated but underlying subclinical health issues that have not been brought to the attention of their primary care physician. The patient has no complaints of insomnia, EDS, or sleep disruption that are attributable to snoring or airflow limitation.

Obstructive Sleep Apnea Syndrome

Apnea is a Greek word that means "without breath." The sleep apnea syndrome is characterized by frequent cessations of breathing during sleep. Physiologically, apnea can be classified into three types: central, obstructive, and mixed [12].

When central sleep apnea (CSA) is diagnosed, it must be pure CSA or at least 80 % of mixed sleep apnea. When most of the events are obstructive or mixed, OSA [13] is diagnosed. The severity of the syndrome, in both OSA and CSA, is primarily determined by the rate of sleep-disordered breathing (SDB) events per hour of sleep (respiratory disturbance index or RDI; apnea–hypopnea index or AHI) and the magnitude of associated oxygen desaturations. As both hypopneas and complete apneas result in arousals from sleep, the distinction between them is not considered important from a severity point of view.

OSA is the most prevalent sleep disorder seen in diagnostic sleep laboratories worldwide, accounting for some 75–80 % of the diagnoses. CSA is considerably less prevalent, except for specific patient populations, such as patients with chronic heart failure or patients with neurological disorders.

Central Sleep Apnea Syndrome

CSA is the cessation of an airflow without any respiratory effort to move air into or out of the lungs. Although the etiology is unknown, there are investigations suggesting that this disorder is related to cardiac problems or central nervous system dysfunction associated with a ventilatory controller mechanism. A PSG in the sleep laboratory similar to the evaluation for OSA is necessary for diagnosis. However, different than the PSG demonstrating OSA, there is an absence of any respiratory effort throughout the duration of the apneic episode for CSA.

The CSA patient suffers from EDS, frequent arousals, and awakenings during sleep or insomnia complaints and/or awakening by shortness of breath.

Obstructive Sleep Apnea Syndromes

OSA is characterized by repetitive episodes of partial (hypopnea) or complete (apnea) upper airway obstruction occurring during sleep.

Sleep apnea literally involves the cessation of breathing on a repeated basis during sleep. This can occur for a brief period of time for a few seconds to longer than a minute, and the frequency can be as much as several hundreds of times during a sleep period.

OSA typically involves an airway obstruction that results in an increased respiratory effort and insufficient ventilation. OSA can involve complete blockage of the upper airway resulting in an apneic episode or partial blockage of the airway resulting in a hypopneic episode. Whereas apnea is complete cessation of airflow, hypopnea is characterized by a 70 % reduction of airflow for >10 s or any reduction in airflow that is associated with either an arousal from sleep or a >3 % arterial oxygen desaturation. Apneas and hypopneas as a result of these varying degrees and locations of upper airway obstructions are regarded as the most common SRBD.

Hypersomnias

Daytime sleepiness, or hypersomnia, is the inability to stay awake and alert during the major waking episodes of the day, resulting in unintended lapses into drowsiness or sleep.

Hypersomnia is a group of disorders in which the primary complaint is daytime sleepiness and in which the cause of the primary symptom is not disturbed nocturnal sleep or misaligned circadian rhythms.

EDS is sleepiness that interferes with activities and quality of life during the waking hours. Typically the individual is unable to remain alert and awake during the hours that are normally regarded as the waking hours for that individual. EDS may be an indication that the individual is suffering from an inadequate amount of sleep, a fragmented or disrupted sleep.

Narcolepsy with Cataplexy

Narcolepsy with cataplexy is primarily characterized by excessive daytime sleepiness. Many of its symptoms are due to an unusual proclivity to transition rapidly from wakefulness into REM sleep and to experience dissociated REM sleep events. A definite history of cataplexy, defined as sudden and transient episodes of loss of muscle tone triggered by emotions, is present.

Narcolepsy Without Cataplexy

Excessive daytime sleepiness in narcolepsy without cataplexy is most typically associated with naps that are refreshing in nature, while nocturnal sleep is normal or moderately disturbed without excessive amounts of sleep.

The two most common types of narcolepsy are that with cataplexy and that without cataplexy. Some individuals who initially do not exhibit cataplexy will subsequently develop such episodes with their narcolepsy.

The multiple sleep latency test (MSLT) is used to assess daytime sleepiness and diagnose narcolepsy.

Circadian Rhythm Sleep Disorders

For optimal sleep, the desired sleep time should match the timing of the circadian rhythm of sleep and wake propensity. Therefore, a recurrent or a chronic pattern of sleep disturbance may result from alterations of the circadian timing system or a misalignment between the timing of the individual's circadian rhythm of sleep propensity and the 24-h social and physical environments.

Circadian rhythm sleep disorders (CRSD) [14] should be included as a possibility when considering a differential diagnosis of individuals who report EDS, insomnia, and impairment of daily functional activities.

Circadian in Latin means "about a day." The human body has an internal timing that demonstrates a circadian rhythm, and one of the more powerful external stimuli for indicating time is the light–dark cycle. Another time indicator for the body is melatonin [15], which is low during the day since light suppresses the secretion of melatonin and increases as the body prepares for the onset of sleep.

The common chronophysiologic characteristic of CRSD is the recurrent asynchrony between the individual's pattern of sleep and what is regarded as society's norm for sleep. With most CRSD cases, the individual has difficulty sleeping at the desired sleep time or when it is required. When there is the desynchronization of the individual's circadian clock relative to the light–dark cycle, CRSD can occur.

Parasomnias

Parasomnias are undesirable physical events or experiences that occur during all sleep stages from entry into sleep to arousals from sleep.

Parasomnias are undesirable and unintended physical and/or subjective experiences that occur as the individual begins to enter into sleep, during sleep, or during arousals from sleep. Included in these disorders are sleep-related movements, emotions, behaviors, dreaming, and functioning of the autonomic nervous system. Parasomnias often take place during arousal and transitions between sleep states when there is reorganization of brain activity, which lends to the belief that the sleep and waking states are not mutually exclusive. The result, therefore, of the overlap of one state with the other is these episodes.

Of the parasomnias, those considered to be disorders of arousal are the most common and can manifest in 4 % of the adult population. Examples of such arousals can include sleepwalking, mumbling, shrieking, disorientation upon awakening, limb paralysis, and uncontrollable eating.

Sleep Movement Disorders

Restless Leg Syndrome

Restless legs syndrome (RLS) [16] is a sensorimotor disorder characterized by a complaint of a strong, nearly irresistible, urge to move the legs. This urge to move is often but not always accompanied by other uncomfortable paresthesias felt deep inside the legs or is a feeling that is simply difficult or impossible to describe.

Episodes of RLS are present mainly when the individual is at rest or during periods of inactivity, and they occur later in the day/evening or as the individual is attempting to initiate sleep. Generally, the experience can have a duration of a few minutes to several hours.

Individuals often describe associated paresthesias or uncomfortable sensations such as jittery or itchy feelings being associated with RLS [17]. The urge to move the legs and the paresthesias can be so unpleasant as to preclude the individual from initiating sleep. It has also been reported that individuals can awaken from sleep because of the RLS episode. Often the individual will relieve these sensations by getting up and walking. It is not uncommon to associate RLS in individuals who demonstrate reduced iron levels along with renal failure.

Periodic Limb Movement Disorder

Periodic limb movement disorder (PLMD) is characterized by periodic episodes of repetitive, highly stereotyped, limb movements that occur during sleep (PLMS) and by clinical sleep disturbance that cannot be accounted for by another primary sleep disorder.

PLMD is characterized by repetitive limb movements that occur during sleep. PLMD can be associated with RLS [17], although PLMD can stand alone as an episode independent of RLS. These periodic episodes of limb movement can result in sleep disturbances[7], although the individual is usually unaware of such partial arousal or awakenings. Even though the disorder is unrecognized by the individual, it is not uncommon for the individual to report a history of EDS and/or insomnia.

PLMD usually displays as extensions of the big toe or flexions of the ankle, knee, or hip, but it can also involve the upper limbs.

Note: The PLMS index must be interpreted in the context of a patient's sleep-related complaint. In adults, normative values higher than the previously accepted value of 5 per hour have been found in studies that did not exclude respiratory event-related arousals (using sensitive respiratory monitoring) and other causes for PLMS. New data suggest a partial overlap of PLMS index values between symptomatic and asymptomatic individuals, emphasizing the importance of clinical context over an absolute cutoff value.

Sleep-Related Leg Cramps

Sleep-related leg cramps are painful sensations caused by sudden and intense involuntary contractions of muscles or muscle groups, usually in the calf of small muscles of the foot, occurring during sleep.

Sleep-related leg cramps are characterized by sudden intense muscle contractions that occur during sleep. Typically, the muscles of the calves or the feet are affected. This disorder has also been known as "charley horse."

These cramps usually occur during sleep, which then result in a disruption of sleep such as an arousal or even an awakening with severe pain. Because of these disruptions to sleep, the individual may report EDS and/or insomnia.

Sleep-Related Bruxism

Sleep bruxism is an oral activity characterized by a repetitive activity (repeated at least three times per episode) in the jaw muscles that generates tooth-grinding sounds and occasionally jaw clenching. Grinding or clenching of the teeth during sleep is usually associated with sleep arousals.

Sleep-related bruxism (SRB) is an oromotor activity characterized by clenching and/or grinding of the teeth during sleep, and it is regarded as a separate entity than bruxism that occurs during the waking hours.

The etiology and pathophysiology of the disorder are unknown. However anxiety and stressful life situations have both been suggested to be risk factors, but more studies are needed in general population to confirm this association. Most SRB events tend to occur in clusters in relation to recurrent arousals (7–14 times per hour of sleep) with transient (3.0 to 10.0 s) reactivation of muscle tone, brain, and heart activities during sleep. According to the reports of children's parents, awareness of tooth-grinding sounds in infants stands at 14–18 %. Findings based on the reports of sleep partners show that 8 % of adults make tooth-grinding sounds, a level that drops to 3 % in older individuals, although this estimate is less precise because of the presence of dentures and habits of sleeping alone.

In dentistry, bruxism is regarded as a mandibular parafunctional activity, whereas in sleep medicine, SRB is considered to be a movement disorder. The patient reports or is aware of tooth-grinding sounds or tooth clenching during sleep. One or more of the following is present: abnormal wear of the teeth, headaches on awakening, jaw muscle discomfort, fatigue, limited mouth opening in the morning, meniscus displacement, jaw pain upon awakening, and masseter muscle hypertrophy.

A dentist's decision to request a sleep laboratory examination may be based on frequent tooth grinding as reported by parents or sleep partners, tooth damage, and orofacial pain (OFP) [18] or headache in relation to sleep [19]. The diagnosis is confirmed by polygraphic recordings of masseter muscle activity and audio–video recordings. Patients with mild sleep bruxism will exhibit more than two jaw muscle contractions per hour of sleep, and patients with moderate-to-severe SRB will exhibit more than four such events per hour of sleep. The differential diagnosis of SRB must exclude the tooth tapping activity and sounds associated with faciomandibular myoclonus. This disorder causes rapid jaw muscle contractions (of less than 0.25-s duration) and is found in 10 % of tooth grinding events. Faciomandibular myoclonus is dominant in REM sleep, and, because it may be associated with sleep-related epilepsy or RBD, a full electroencephalographic examination is recommended.

Children may exhibit various tics during sleep, including throat grunting, enuresis, and sleep talking, and these also have to be excluded in the diagnostic process. SDB such as sleep apnea in children or in older individuals also must be verified in the sleep laboratory. The persistence of wakeful dyskinetic movement (dystonia, tremor, chorea, and dyskinesia) is also possible, but it is rarely concomitant with sleep bruxism.

Sleep Disorders Associated with Other Medical Conditions

Numerous medical conditions affect sleep or are affected by sleep. The list is a small number of medical disorders that may be of particular importance to sleep specialists.

Pain and Sleep

Insomnia, lack of sleep, and other sleep disorders intensify the pain conditions. Also pain can cause poor sleep, loss of sleep, and a reduction in an adequate number of hours of sleep that only continues to perpetuate the vicious pain cycle. Therefore, improving sleep can cause pain relief or reduction.

Studies have demonstrated that chronic pain can be present in 11–29 % of the adult population and that 50–90 % of these individuals can indicate that their sleep is adversely affected by their pain [20].

Sleep loss, specifically 4-h and REM-type sleep, is associated with hyperalgesia the following day. There is a bidirectional relationship between the loss of sleep and pain; that is, the loss of sleep impacts pain levels, and pain levels can reduce the amount of sleep [21].

In patients with osteoarthritis, improvement of sleep latency and sleep efficiency was analgesic when compared to control subjects.

Dentists encounter a number of painful conditions, and it is imperative that the loss or the lack of sleep be considered in the overall management plan for the painful condition. In addition, it is essential that an understanding of the relationship between pain and its relationship to the sleep state be considered when planning for the management of each situation and condition.

Orofacial Pain

Dentists deal with dental and oral pain, so they have more interest in the head and neck pain, including headaches. As with pain in general, these conditions are frequently associated with some type of sleep disruption. It is difficult to determine which came first, the pain or the sleep problem.

Temporomandibular Disorders

The occurrence of temporomandibular disorders (TMDs) in conjunction with poor sleep may be associated with MFP and/or bruxism that occurs during sleep and/or waking hours.

Myofacial Pain

Muscle pain is a common finding among patients with poor sleep. The patients with muscle pain are most likely to have insomnia. However, not all patients with poor sleep will have muscle pain or muscle tenderness when palpated. Sleep disturbance is a common finding in myofacial pain (MFP) patients.

Patients with lack of sleep and sleep breathing disorders may suffer from fibromyalgia (FM). One study demonstrated that greater than 50 % of subjects diagnosed with FM also experienced chronic fatigue. The FM patient will have the presence of multiple tender points that have been anatomically mapped, and the presence of these is a factor in determining the risk for this condition. MFP and FM are related, and their coexistence as well as the relationship to sleep disorders are important to recognize.

Trigeminal and Glossopharyngeal Neuralgia

This particular facial neuralgia is paroxysmal in nature and is precipitated by function or touch. The attacks are often unilateral, and they are described as sharp or electric-like and usually brief and unpredictable. The interesting fact related to this pain and sleep relationship is that the attacks do not occur during sleep.

Temporal Arteritis (TA)

Also known as giant cell arteritis, this is a painful headache-like condition with throbbing around the area of the temporal artery. The patient may have pain in the masticatory [22] muscles associated with chewing. The pain will frequently be worse at night and may be exaggerated by resting the head on a pillow. Because of the serious nature of this type of pain, immediate attention to the treatment should be initiated.

Toothache

Anecdotally, toothache is one of the OFP conditions that can interfere significantly with sleep. Patients with acute pulpitis or apical periodontitis often report awakenings and lack of sleep due to pain. Epidemiologic studies have, indeed, substantiated the influence of toothaches on sleep. Periodontal pain after adjustment of orthodontic archwires is reported to have little influence on sleep.

Idiopathic Atypical Odontalgia

This type of OFP is what appears to the patient as being an odontogenic pain, but it is without any distinct or obvious dental pathology. The pain is typically more prevalent in the maxillary posterior teeth, and it does not resolve with the use of local anesthesia. Because the pain is continuous and a cause is frequently elusive, the patient may become depressed or have increased stress, which in turn may lead to insomnia.

These patients will usually report that they will awaken with this pain, but they do not awaken because of the pain. The treatment of this condition is generally responsive to a low-dose regimen of tricyclic antidepressant medication.

Headache Disorders

Headache and sleep disorders are the most prevalent conditions seen in clinical practice [23]. As with other painful conditions, headaches can be related to sleep disturbances. Also similar to other pain, the headaches frequently will not resolve unless the sleep disorder is also addressed. As such, sleep may both provoke as well as relieve headaches.

In particular, chronic daily and morning headaches are indicators of a probable sleep disorder. These encompass SRBD, insomnia, circadian rhythm disorders, and parasomnias. The most frequently reported headaches that are related to a sleep disorder are migraine, cluster, and muscle tension type.

Headache seems to be more common in snorers as compared to non-snorers. Habitual snoring is also more prevalent in chronic daily headache patients than in those with episodic headache. Insomnia can lead to headache, and the severity of headache is related directly to the degree of insomnia. Because insomnia is the most common sleep complaint relative to sleep disorders, it is found to occur in one-half to two-thirds of headache patients.

In cluster headache, the presence of OSA is 8.4 times that of the normal population. When the patient is over 40 years of age and has an increased body mass index (BMI), the odds ratio increases. Accordingly, the risk decreases with a lower BMI and when the patient is less than 40 years old.

In the ICSD-2, the most common headaches that are sleep related are the following: cluster, migraine, tension type, and paroxysmal hemicrania. Of the patients who had headache, 53 % were diagnosed with OSA.

When a patient reports temporal or tension-type headaches on awakening, the dentist must assess for SDB or sleep bruxism [24] because these are frequently related complaints. Dentists should gather the patient's and the sleep partner's reports of snoring, cessation of breathing, and sleepiness by using the Epworth Sleepiness Scale (ESS) questionnaire.

Sleep-related headaches are a group of unilateral or bilateral headaches of varying severity and duration that occur during sleep or upon awakening from sleep. Sleep medicine recognizes the association that may exist for some individuals relative to sleep disorders and various headache disorders, including migraine, cluster, chronic daily, awakening or morning, and tension-type headaches. As compared to the general population, individuals with headaches demonstrate a two- to eightfold greater risk for sleep disorders, and the most common sleep disorder associated with headache subjects is insomnia.

It has been suggested that the neuroanatomy of the hypothalamus and the neurophysiological mechanisms involving the secretions of serotonin and melatonin may be contributory to the comorbidity of sleep disorders and headaches. Relative to cluster headache, melatonin secretion may be impaired in those individuals.

Modifications of sleep hygiene such as sleep loss, sleep disturbance, and even oversleeping have been identified as the most common precipitating factors of migraine and tension-type headaches. Studies demonstrated a significant increase in SRBD with cluster headache subjects.

Migraine attacks can also be reported during the sleep period because about half of such attacks are reported to occur between 4 and 9 AM. Migraine attacks mainly occur in relation to REM sleep, although they sometimes occur during deep sleep (stages (N3) and (N4)). Patients may also report the occurrence of cluster headaches during REM sleep; such headaches are unilaterally periocular or temporal in nature and accompanied by autonomic reaction. A rare form of sleep-related headache is the hypnic headache, which occurs at sleep onset. The hypnic headache is mainly found in older patients and tends to be bilateral.

The review suggests that (1) chronic daily headache, and especially "morning headache," is a particular, though nonspecific, indicator for sleep disorders; (2) the identification and management of a primary sleep disorder in the presence of headache may improve or resolve the headache (headache secondary to primary sleep disorder); (3) headache patients exhibit a high incidence of sleep disturbance which might trigger or exacerbate headache; and (4) such primary headache may improve with regulation of sleep. These findings argue for screening and management of sleep disturbance among headache patients.

Fibromyalgia (FM)

According to the 1990 American College of Rheumatology consensus criteria, FM is characterized by widespread pain of at least 3-month duration and muscle tenderness, lack of sleep, headaches, anxiety, and mood alteration [25].

FM is a syndrome described by multiple tender point sites and long-standing musculoskeletal pain that is usually diffuse. The criteria for FM established by the American College of Rheumatology states that there must be a widespread distribution above and below the waist of musculoskeletal pain occurring for a minimum of 3 months along with 11 or more of the 18 recognized tender points. The prevalence of FM is the second most common rheumatological disorder after osteoarthritis. It is reported that more than 80–96 % of patients with FM may also suffer from poor sleep quality (also reported as a sensation of unrefreshing sleep) and TMDs or pain.

The sleep-related brain activity termed alpha–delta sleep is no longer considered a pathognomonic finding in these patients. Clinicians making a differential diagnosis in these patients must exclude periodic limb movement during sleep and SDB.

Many individuals with the FM syndrome also experience sleep disturbances that can result in feeling tired, unrefreshed sleep, reduced cognitive function, and early awakening from sleep. It has been found that most subjects with FM experienced microarousals and an electroencephalographic alpha–delta or alpha–NREM anomaly that interrupts the deep stage (N4) restorative level of sleep. This EEG anomaly, though, may not be specific to FM as it has also been found in individuals who did not have FM complaints.

Gastroesophageal Reflux

Sleep-related gastroesophageal reflux also known as heartburn is characterized by regurgitation of stomach contents into the esophagus during sleep. This sleep disorder may result in a pain that is usually located substernal, but it may also manifest in the area of the throat.

Subjective Self-Assessment

Although this type of self-assessment methodology does not provide objective physiologic data that measure wake/sleep periods of the patient, it does allow for a lower cost method to easily acquire at least some patient-based information that can be correlated with the patient's history and clinical examination.

Epworth Sleepiness Scale

The most frequently used instrument is ESS, which was developed in 1991. It has been demonstrated to identify degrees of sleepiness, and the results are considered to be within acceptable limits for test–retest reliability. The eight questions of the ESS query the individual about his or her subjective reporting of sleepiness relative to his or her expectation of dozing in eight different situations.

In using a scale of 0–3, where 0 indicates no chance of dozing, 1 indicates a slight chance, 2 indicates a moderate chance, and 3 indicates a high chance, a total maximum score of 24 is possible. Investigations have shown that a score of 10 or 11 is considered to be the upper parameter for normal. While higher scores correlate with sleep disorders, it has also been shown that scores also improve relative to the efficacy of management of SRBD.

Although the ESS is attractive via its simplicity and ease of administration, the instrument does have its limitations, including not taking into account the individual's age, acuteness of sleep pathology, medical conditions, or use of pharmaceutics. Thus, the ESS is best when it is employed to be an adjunct to the patient history and clinical examination.

Clinical Assessment

As defined by the American Academy of Sleep Medicine (AASM), there are four levels (I–IV) of sleep studies from which an objective-based assessment is made. A level I study is regarded as the most accepted study for the assessment and treatment of OSA. The four levels are differentiated as per the number of simultaneously recorded physiological signals as well as whether or not the sleep study was attended by a sleep technologist.

Polysomnography

A polysomnography (PSG) is an overnight sleep study attended by a sleep technologist during which at least seven different physiological signals are measured, and it is a level I study. The PSG is considered to be the "gold standard" in sleep medicine relative to objective-based sleep studies. The study is usually conducted in a sleep laboratory/center type of facility with trained staffs to ensure proper placement of the necessary sensors as well as recognize and address any displacement of sensors as needed during the study.

The physiologic parameters measured during a PSG include simultaneous and continuous monitoring of at least brain wave activity, eye movements, muscle activity of the legs and mandible, body position, heart rate and rhythm, blood pressure, snoring, and respiratory activity that includes breathing patterns and oxygen saturation. Analysis of the data from these various measurements can reveal sleep disorder activities such as apnea. A summary of the entire PSG data can be reflected in a graphic form called a hypnogram which provides a comprehensive glimpse of sleep architecture relative to stages of sleep.

The raw data are scored into different sleep stages and physiologic activities in accordance with standardized criteria, and a sleep physician interprets the study results, reviews the patient history and clinical examination data, and subsequently prepares a sleep study report of outcomes and recommendations. Most common sleep disorders can be assessed with a PSG, including SRBD. Effectiveness of treatment methods can also be achieved with a PSG.

PSG performed in a sleep laboratory involves continuous overnight recording of a minimum of 12 channels of sleep- and breathing-related measurements, such as EEG, electrooculogram, electromyogram, nasal airflow (preferably measured by nasal pressure cannula), oral airflow (thermistor), respiratory effort, oxygen saturation, body position, and electrocardiogram. Recordings require manual scoring of the events by trained sleep technologists and interpretation of the results by sleep medicine physicians, taking into account the clinical context. The examinations monitor the occurrence of apneas (complete cessation of airflow for 10 s or more) and hypopneas (reduction in amplitude of airflow or thoracoabdominal wall movement for 10 s or more with an accompanying oxygen desaturation of at least 3 % and/or associated arousals). OSA is defined as a total of more than five events per hour of sleep. Notably, variations exist in scoring definitions, especially for hypopneas.

The severity of sleep apnea is assessed with the AHI, although other factors such as the degree of oxygen desaturation and the extent of sleep fragmentation are important for the clinical interpretation of OSA severity. Some laboratories report an RDI, which often incorporates all respiratory events (beyond apneas and hypopneas), although the definition for this score may vary.

Generally, diagnosis of OSA can be based on a single night of testing, although night-to-night variability in results should be considered, especially if test results are negative for a patient with high clinical risk of OSA. Apparent variability in the severity of OSA may result from a number of factors, including differences in sleeping position, alcohol use, prior sleep debt, sleep efficiency, and sleep stage distribution. Furthermore, variation in the definitions and scoring of the respiratory events can also significantly alter the AHI. The major limitations of PSG are that it is expensive and labor intensive, and thus waiting lists for the procedure tend to be very long.

Multiple Sleep Latency Test

An MSLT is commonly used to measure daytime sleepiness. The MSLT consists of a series of four to five 20-min daytime naps during 2-h intervals at a sleep laboratory/center, and the test often lasts 7–8 h. In addition, the test is to begin 1.5–3 h after awakening from an overnight PSG. Similar to the PSG, sensors are placed by a trained sleep technologist in order to measure brain wave activity, eye movements, muscle activity of the mandible, and cardiac activity. There are standardized conditions under which the MSLT is performed, including the instruction to the patient, such as "Please lie quietly, assume a comfortable position, keep your eyes closed, and try to fall asleep."

The physiological data outcomes demonstrate the amount of time it takes for the individual to initiate sleep (i.e., sleep latency) and to attain the different stages of sleep during each nap. The final scoring for the MSLT is the averaged times of sleep latency for the series of naps. An MSLT score of greater than 10 min is considered normal and less than 5 min is regarded as generally indicating the presence of a sleep disorder. Individuals who demonstrate a quick onset of REM sleep are also more likely to have a sleep disorder. Often the MSLT is the instrument of choice to definitively diagnose narcolepsy [26] or idiopathic hypersomnia. The MSLT can also be used to document outcomes of treatment. Residual sleepiness can also be demonstrated for those individuals who do not report sleepiness after undergoing treatment.

In and of itself, the MSLT is not regarded as an accurate means to differentiate pathologic sleep disorders. Practice parameters for the clinical application of the MSLT have been published by the AASM.

Maintenance of Wakefulness Test

A maintenance of wakefulness test (MWT) is commonly used to measure the alertness of an individual during the waking hours. The MWT can also be employed to assess a sleep disorder patient's response to treatment. Whereas the MSLT determines whether or not an individual can initiate sleep sooner than what is regarded as a normal amount of time, the MWT determines whether or not an individual can stay awake for what is regarded as a normal amount of time.

Similar to the MSLT, sensors are placed by a trained sleep technologist in order to measure brain wave activity, eye movements, muscle activity of the mandible, and cardiac activity, and subsequently there is a series of four to five 20-min daytime naps during 2-h intervals at a sleep laboratory/center. Although there are also similar standardized conditions under which the MWT is performed, the significant procedural difference of the MWT from the MSLT is with the instruction to the patient, "Please sit still and remain awake for as long as possible." Look directly ahead of you, and do not look directly at the light.

The physiological data outcomes demonstrate the ability of an individual to stay awake. The final scoring for the MWT is the averaged times of wakefulness for the series. An MWT score of 8 min or more is considered normal, whereas abnormal would be an average of initiating sleep in less than 8 min. If the individual does not fall asleep in 40 min, then the test is terminated.

Practice parameters for the clinical application of the MSLT have been published by the AASM.

With a heightened awareness in sleep disorders relative to public safety, the MWT is acknowledged by the Federal Aviation Administration as a method of assessing effectiveness of treatment for EDS, thereby affording the ability to the aviation medical examiners to reissue an airman medical certificate for commercial airline pilots.

As with the other assessment instruments, test outcomes must be viewed in light of the patient history and clinical examination. Also, it has been shown that there is poor correlation between the ESS, MSLT, and MWT.

Sleep Apnea Management/Treatment

Behavioral Management

Behavioral treatment involves the abstinence from alcohol and sedatives in the early evening. The intake of alcohol selectively reduces the muscle tone of the upper airway and increases the frequency of abnormal breathing during sleep. Alcohol also prolongs apnea by delaying arousal. Behavioral methods also include training patients to sleep in a lateral position if upper airway obstruction is present only during sleep in the supine position. Weight reduction in a patient without anatomical risk factors can often eliminate OSA.

Medical Treatment

Patients with OSA, snoring, or upper airway resistance syndrome (UARS) will benefit primarily from positive airway pressure (PAP) [27–30]. However, the patient's compliance is a major issue in this therapy, which frustrates the sleep specialists and patient's bed partner.

The PAP device produces a positive pressurized airflow that is delivered to the patient via a mask over the face.

There are three primary types of PAP modes: (1) continuous positive airway pressure (CPAP), (2) bilevel positive airway pressure (BiPAP) [31], and (3) autoadjusting positive airway pressure (APAP). A fourth mode receiving some attention is the expiratory pressure relief mode (flexible CPAP).

There is a significant amount of published literature about PAP therapy. The purpose of this chapter is to present an emphasis on PAP therapy as it relates to the adult population with SRBD, in particular OSA.

Medical treatment involves the use of CPAP [32]; it is a device that controls apnea by providing a stream of air, under slight pressure, through a tube into the nasal passage. This positive air pressure acts as a splint holding the tissues in the back of the throat open to prevent collapse. Use of this device requires a sleep study to determine the proper pressure to use.

This treatment is regarded by most as the first fine of treatment in patients with moderate to severe OSA. This generally means patients with more than 20 episodes of apnea or hypopnea per hour with associated oxygen desaturations. However, patient's compliance with CPAP is approximately 50 %. Many patients therefore go untreated. Side effects reported by patients include irritation related to the nasal mask, nasal congestion [33], occasional rhinorrhea, and feelings of claustrophobia.

Besides effectiveness for management of moderate to severe OSA cases, PAP therapy may be effective for the management of mild OSA. However, there is a greater propensity for those with mild OSA to demonstrate less adherence (compliance) to PAP therapy. It is important for even those individuals with mild OSA to know that there exists the increased risk for cardiovascular issues, such as HT.

The individuals with mild OSA or even primary (benign) snoring may not find appealing the alternative treatment options that include either surgical intervention of the upper airway tissues or use of an OA [34]. The remaining possible conservative options include weight loss, sleep positional changes, sleep hygiene modifications, or other alternative therapies.

As with other areas of medical care, there are Medicare guidelines for PAP therapy reimbursement, which can serve as references for the indications of PAP therapy. If there is an AHI of 5–14 episodes/h that represents mild OSA, then there must also be symptoms or signs of significant impairment. Impairments that qualify include EDS, HT, insomnia, mood disorders, and cardiovascular issues. These impairments are not required for individuals with an AHI of 15 or more episodes per hour that represent moderate to severe OSA.

The effectiveness of PAP therapy for each individual diagnosed with OSA is assessed during an attended PSG or sleep study. During the PSG visit, the type of PAP mask interface and the level of airflow pressure effective for managing the OSA are established. This determination may be done during a second sleep study, also known as a two-night study, or it may be performed during the latter portion of a single-sleep study, also known as a split-night study.

Dental Appliances

OA therapy has been used for the management of sleep apnea, snoring, and upper airway resistance since the early 1930s [35].

Dental appliances in the treatment of OSA are of three classes. One type attempts to push the soft palate with a distal extension from a palate plate. This neither has nor found wide acceptance due to gagging and the uncertainty of maintaining hypopharyngeal width during sleep. The second class of appliances is designed to act directly on the tongue by holding it forward by means of negative pressure from an anterior suction bulb or proprioceptive reminder. The tongue-retaining device (TRD) is the most successful of these appliances, especially in the elimination of snoring. The third group of appliances repositions the mandible in a more protrusive position and has general acceptance as being the most effective device in the elimination of both snoring and OSA. Both these TRD and MAD are designed to reduce the upper airway obstruction.

Standards of practice guidelines relative to the use and effectiveness of OA therapy for OSA and snoring were first published in 1995 by the AASM case studies comprising the evidence on which those initial clinical guidelines were based. The AASM guidelines document noted that OA therapy can be considered as a first-line treatment option for the management of mild OSA and simple snoring and also as a second-line treatment option for moderate OSA after unsuccessful attempts with other treatment options. Following the publication of these guidelines, significant research-based findings pertaining to OA therapy have been published [36, 37].

In 2006, the AASM published two documents that further recognized OA therapy as a medical device option for the management of OSA and snoring: (1) an evidence-based review of literature regarding OA therapy in sleep medicine and (2) a practice parameter update. Scientific literature published since 1995 comprised the evidence on which the current practice parameters were based. The updated practice parameters indicate that OA therapy is now an option for patients with mild to moderate sleep apnea and who prefer this method of treatment as opposed to using CPAP. In addition, OA therapy may be utilized in patients with severe sleep apnea who (1) are unable to tolerate CPAP, (2) have failed surgery, or (3) are primary (benign) snorers (i.e., snoring without apnea).

OAs have also been reviewed by the US Food and Drug Administration (FDA), and OAs are regarded as class II medical devices. The FDA document states that special controls apply to these devices, and they are deemed to be medical devices appropriate for the treatment of OSA. As such, OAs marketed to the public for the treatment/management of OSA and snoring are required to have a 510 k or premarket notification clearance in order to be commercially available.

The mechanism by which these appliances work appears simple. Mandibular advancement splints prevent the tongue from collapsing against the posterior pharyngeal wall nocturnally. This is achieved by mechanical means in that the origin and insertion of genioglossus are at the hyoid bone and mandibular symphyseal region, respectively. Thus, by advancing the mandible, the tongue is held in a more anterior position at night. Elevation of the hyoid bone in an anterosuperior direction is therefore the desired radiographic modification. A second consideration given by Lowe et al. is that, in man, voluntary passive opening of the mandible produces definite enhancement of genioglossus EMG through activation of receptors located in the temporomandibular joint. Because the contraction of the genioglossus opens the airway, airway obstruction may be prevented.

Despite considerable variation in the design of these appliances, the desired effects are remarkably consistent. Snoring is reduced and often eliminated in almost all patients who use OAs. Theoretical complications of long-term use of mandibular advancement splints include temporomandibular joint dysfunction.

However, intermittent forward positions of the mandible have yet to be shown to produce irreversible TMJ dysfunction as a consequence. Limited follow-up data indicate that oral discomfort is a common but tolerable side effect and that dental and mandibular complications appear to be uncommon.

Surgical Treatment

Surgical Therapy for OSA

A surgical solution to OSA, if successful, eliminates any question of compliance.

The surgical approach to SDB continues to evolve. Many surgical approaches have emerged, including tracheostomy, uvulopalatopharyngoplasty (UPPP), laser-assisted UPPP (LAUP), septoplasty, orthognathic surgery, and radiofrequency volumetric tissue reduction (RFVTR) ("somnoplasty" or "coblation"). Most recently, palatal implants have been developed and marketed as treatments for sleep apnea. The effects of bariatric surgery on adult sleep apnea have also been investigated. However, outside of tracheostomy and jaw advancement, telegnathic surgery remains the most accepted successful surgical therapy for OSA at this time [38].

In an extensive search for relevant studies of randomized trials of UPPP treatment for sleep apnea, the Cochrane investigators found eight studies, totaling 412 participants. Surgical treatment of SDB has been so poorly evaluated in the literature that it cannot be recommended to patients as a first-line treatment option. A common problem is that the surgical literature continues to define "success" on the basis of reduction in RDI by 50 % and not on a more strict definition.

UPPP and LAUP

UPPP is the most commonly performed and best studied of the surgical procedures used to treat sleep apnea. In this procedure, redundant soft palate and pharyngeal tissues, uvula, and tonsils are removed. Potential complications include velopharyngeal insufficiency, stenosis, and dysphagia. Because of problems with UPPP, several variations on this theme have emerged, including the uvulopalatal flap and laser-assisted uvula palatoplasty (LAUP for the uninitiated). Unfortunately, there simply is no sufficient evidence that these procedures are beneficial for patients with sleep apnea.

Radiofrequency Volumetric Tissue Reduction

RFVTR applied to the palate ("somnoplasty") was originally investigated as a less painful treatment option for SDB than UPPP. This procedure has largely been abandoned as treatment for sleep apnea, though it is occasionally used primarily for snoring.

Oral and Maxillofacial Surgery (Telegnathic Surgery)

When applying the basic orthognathic surgical technique for the purpose of effecting airway expansion in patients with OSA, the correct terminology is "telegnathic surgery." This term differentiates this procedure from that performed for correction of dentofacial deformities, as the purpose of this surgery is instead focused on airway expansion.

In a recent review of oral and maxillofacial surgery, Prinsell et al. concluded, "MMA" (maxillomandibular advancement surgery) for OSA surgery is a highly successful and potentially definitive primary single-staged surgery that may result in a significant reduction in OSA syndrome-related health risks, as well as financial savings for the health care system." Li reaches the same conclusion: MMA surgery is the most effective procedure for OSA. In four studies including a total of 214 patients who had MMA the (surgically defined) success rate was 96–100 %. MMA results in enlargement of the entire upper airway.

Jaw advancement surgery is better tolerated and has a far more significant and beneficial effect than most airway soft tissue surgical procedures and may produce beneficial effects on nocturnal breathing. Excellent long-term (5-year) results have been noted in patients who do not gain weight postoperatively, and favorable effects on quality of life following telegnathic surgery have been documented.

Application of this procedure to the pediatric population using distraction osteogenesis techniques continues to advance, as new and modified distraction devices continue to evolve. Distraction osteogenesis offers the treating surgeon the ability to "titrate" the degree of advancement with the amount of airway expansion needed to resolve the airway problem. Rapid maxillary expansion has been shown to have very favorable effects in the growing child on improvement (and often elimination) of OSA.

Telegnathic surgery is appropriate when there are ill effects from the use of MRAs on the temporomandibular joints, occlusion, lack of compliance to an OA, failure of previous soft tissue surgical procedures, and other structural anomalies present, such as in the hypoplastic or constricted maxilla.

The surgical methods to eliminate OSA include reduction of the inferior turbinate bones, adenoidectomy (nasopharyngeal involvement), UPPP, tonsillectomy (oropharyngeal involvement), genioglossal and hyoid advancement (hypopharyngeal involvement), bimaxillary advancement, and tracheostomy. UPPP is curative in less than 50 % of patients. LAUP has recently been introduced as an outpatient treatment for snoring.

UPPP enlarges the oropharynx and reduces the collapsibility of the upper airway. Patients with a narrow oropharynx relative to tongue size have a good response to UPPP.

Surgical treatment of OSA by MMA should be restricted to patients with a retrognathic dolichofacial type combined with pharyngeal narrowing. The maxilla and mandible must both be advanced at least 10 mm to ensure success. In severe instances of OSA that are life threatening, the ultimate treatment is tracheostomy. This procedure completely bypasses the upper airway and thus all upper airway obstruction. The procedure is, however, usually used as the last option in the treatment of OSA.

Conclusion

Understanding sleep and the processes related to it is important because it helps in understanding the dynamics of sleep disorders; since the use of OA for management of OSA is recognized as an acceptable treatment option, the dentist now has an increasing role in the recognition of a patient who may be at risk for a sleep disorder. The dentist does not have to understand the complex neurologic and neurochemical relationships that present with sleep, but it is prudent to have an understanding of the basics, the knowledge of the relevant aspects of sleep, and the ability to recognize how normal sleep may become altered. This understanding allows the dentist to have the foundational knowledge to explain certain aspects of sleep to patients who wish to have a better appreciation of their sleep and why disruption of it is occurring.

In addition, understanding sleep and sleep disorders will enable the dentist to better communicate with physicians regarding a patient who may have sleep disorders. For the sake of the patient, the dentist should have an ever-increasing awareness of medical issues relative to their patients.

It is not necessary for the dentist to determine the specific sleep disorder. More importantly, it is helpful if the dentist can recognize symptoms that may indicate the need for a more appropriate referral.

Acknowledgement The author would like to thank Dr. George Zureikat MD for his recordings of sleep patterns to be used in this chapter.

Conflict of Interest None declared.

References

1. Khan F, Hazin R, Han Y. Apneic disorders associated with heart failure: pathophysiology and clinical management. South Med J. 2010;103(1):44–50.
2. Ross SD, Sheinhait IA, Harrison KJ, Kvasz M, Connelly JE, Shea SA, et al. Systematic review and meta-analysis of the literature regarding the diagnosis of sleep apnea. Sleep. 2000;23(4):519–32.
3. Morin CM, Rodrigue S, Ivers H. Role of stress, arousal, and coping skills in primary insomnia. Psychosom Med. 2003;65(2):259–67.
4. Mitler MM, Gujavarty KS, Browman CP. Maintenance of wakefulness test: a polysomnographic technique for evaluation treatment efficacy in patients with excessive somnolence. Electroencephalogr Clin Neurophysiol. 1982;53(6):658–61.
5. Johns MW. Sensitivity and specificity of the multiple sleep latency test (MSLT), the maintenance of wakefulness test and the Epworth sleepiness scale: failure of the MSLT as a gold standard. J Sleep Res. 2000;9(1):5–11.
6. Sangal RB, Mitler MM, Sangal JM. Subjective sleepiness ratings (Epworth sleepiness scale) do not reflect the same parameter of sleepiness as objective sleepiness (maintenance of wakefulness test) in patients with narcolepsy. Clin Neurophysiol. 1999;110(12):2131–5.
7. Loureiro CC, Drummond M, Winck JC, Almeida J. Clinical and polysomnographic characteristics of patients with REM sleep disordered breathing. Rev Port Pneumol. 2009;15(5):847–57.

8. Roepke SK, Ancoli-Israel S. Sleep disorders in the elderly. Indian J Med Res. 2010; 131:302–10.
9. Wise MS. Objective measures of sleepiness and wakefulness: application to the real world? J Clin Neurophysiol. 2006;23(1):39–49.
10. Kanathur N, Harrington J, Lee-Chiong T. Circadian rhythm sleep disorders. Clin Chest Med. 2010;31(2):319–25.
11. Castriotta RJ, Atanasov S, Wilde MC, Masel BE, Lai JM, Kuna ST. Treatment of sleep disorders after traumatic brain injury. J Clin Sleep Med. 2009;5(2):137–44.
12. White DP. Sleep apnea. Proc Am Thorac Soc. 2006;3(1):124–8.
13. McNicholas WT, Ryan S. Obstructive sleep apnoea syndrome: translating science to clinical practice. Respirology. 2006;11(2):136–44.
14. Silva EJ, Wang W, Ronda JM, Wyatt JK, Duffy JF. Circadian and wake-dependent influences on subjective sleepiness, cognitive throughput, and reaction time performance in older and young adults. Sleep. 2010;33(4):481–90.
15. Cajochen C, Kräuchi K, Wirz-Justice A. Role of melatonin in the regulation of human circadian rhythms and sleep. J Neuroendocrinol. 2003;15(4):432–7.
16. Chahine LM, Chemali ZN. Restless legs syndrome: a review. CNS Spectr. 2006;11(7):511–20.
17. Michaud M, Chabli A, Lavigne G, Montplaisir J. Arm restlessness in patients with restless legs syndrome. Mov Disord. 2000;15(2):289–93.
18. Wong MC, McMillan AS, Zheng J, Lam CL. The consequences of orofacial pain symptoms: a population-based study in Hong Kong. Community Dent Oral Epidemiol. 2008;36(5):417–24.
19. Dodick DW, Eross EJ, Parish JM, Silber M. Clinical, anatomical, and physiologic relationship between sleep and headache. Headache. 2003;43(3):282–92.
20. Smith MT, Perlis ML, Smith MS, Giles DE, Carmody TP. Sleep quality and presleep arousal in chronic pain. J Behav Med. 2000;23(1):1–13.
21. Pilowsky I, Crettenden I, Townley M. Sleep disturbance in pain clinic patients. Pain. 1985;23(1):27–33.
22. Bertoli E, de Leeuw R, Schmidt JE, Okeson JP, Carlson CR. Prevalence and impact of post-traumatic stress disorder symptoms in patients with masticatory muscle or temporomandibular joint pain: differences and similarities. J Orofac Pain. 2007;21(2):107–19.
23. Rains JC, Poceta JS. Headache and sleep disorders: review and clinical implications for headache management. Headache. 2006;46(9):1344–63.
24. Bader GG, Kampe T, Tagdae T, Karlsson S, Blomqvist M. Descriptive physiological data on a sleep bruxism population. Sleep. 1997;20(11):982–90.
25. Morin CM, Gibson D, Wade J. Self-reported sleep and mood disturbance in chronic pain patients. Clin J Pain. 1998;14(4):311–4.
26. Parkes JD, Chen SY, Clift SJ, Dahlitz MJ, Dunn G. The clinical diagnosis of the narcoleptic syndrome. J Sleep Res. 1998;7(1):41–52.
27. Loube DI, Gay PC, Strohl KP, Pack AI, White DP, Collop NA. Indications for positive airway pressure treatment of adult obstructive sleep apnea patients: a consensus statement. Chest. 1999;115(3):863–6.
28. Sanders MH, Montserrat JM, Farré R, Givelber RJ. Positive pressure therapy: a perspective on evidence-based outcomes and methods of application. Proc Am Thorac Soc. 2008;5(2):161–72.
29. Weaver TE, Grunstein RR. Adherence to continuous positive airway pressure therapy: the challenge to effective treatment. Proc Am Thorac Soc. 2008;5(2):173–8.
30. Barnes M, McEvoy RD, Banks S, Tarquinio N, Murray CG, Vowles N, et al. Efficacy of positive airway pressure and oral appliance in mild to moderate obstructive sleep apnea. Am J Respir Crit Care Med. 2004;170(6):656–64.
31. Kushida CA, Littner MR, Hirshkowitz M, Morgenthaler TI, Alessi CA, Bailey D, et al. Practice parameters for the use of continuous and bilevel positive airway pressure devices to treat adult patients with sleep-related breathing disorders. Sleep. 2006;29(3):375–80.

32. Redline S, Adams N, Strauss ME, Roebuck T, Winters M, Rosenberg C. Improvement of mild sleep-disordered breathing with CPAP compared with conservative therapy. Am J Respir Crit Care Med. 1998;157(3 Pt 1):858–65.
33. Sugiura T, Noda A, Nakata S, Yasuda Y, Soga T, Miyata S, et al. Influence of nasal resistance on initial acceptance of continuous positive airway pressure in treatment for obstructive sleep apnea syndrome. Respiration. 2007;74(1):56–60.
34. Ferguson KA, Cartwright R, Rogers R, Schmidt-Nowara W. Oral appliances for snoring and obstructive sleep apnea: a review. Sleep. 2006;29(2):244–62.
35. Hoekema A, Stegenga B, De Bont LG. Efficacy and co-morbidity of oral appliances in the treatment of obstructive sleep apnea-hypopnea: a systematic review. Crit Rev Oral Biol Med. 2004;15(3):137–55.
36. Kushida CA, Morgenthaler TI, Littner MR, Alessi CA, Bailey D, Coleman J, et al. Practice parameters for the treatment of snoring and obstructive sleep apnea with oral appliances: an update for 2005. Sleep. 2006;29(2):240–3.
37. Lim J, Lasserson TJ, Fleetham J, Wright J. Oral appliances for obstructive sleep apnoea. Cochrane Database Syst Rev. 2006;1, CD004435.
38. Sundaram S, Bridgman SA, Lim J, Lasserson TJ. Surgery for obstructive sleep apnoea. Cochrane Database Syst Rev. 2005;4, CD001004.

Chapter 6
Local Anesthesia in the Orofacial Region

Thomas M. Halaszynski

Introduction

Local anesthesia involves the injection or application of an anesthetic drug to a specific area of the body, as opposed to the entire body and brain as typically occurs during general anesthesia (GA). The injection of local anesthetic agents (regional dental anesthesia) in the skin and mucous membranes is one of the most frequently for performed for minor surgical maneuvers for oral and maxillofacial procedures. Depending on the technique employed, regional dental anesthesia can be divided into component parts. Local anesthesia in the dental arena (otherwise known as "Novocain") consists of dental injection(s) that "numbs" the mouth in preparation for dental procedures and oral surgery. The injection(s) may follow the painting of the gums with a topical anesthetic that numbs the oral tissues so that discomfort is minimized while local anesthesia is administered. Patients may use just local anesthesia for their orofacial procedures or they may use it in conjunction with nitrous oxide, intravenous (IV) sedation, or GA. Regardless of the choice, local anesthesia is usually always administered prior invasive to oral procedures and maxillofacial surgery.

A local anesthetic is a drug that causes reversible loss of sensory and/or motor function due to blockage of anesthesia conduction resulting in loss of nociception. When local anesthesia is used on specific nerve pathways (nerve block), effects of analgesia (loss of pain sensation) and paralysis (loss of muscle power) can be achieved. Local anesthetics used clinically belong to one of the two classes: amino amide and amino ester local anesthetics. The synthetic local anesthetics used clinically are structurally related cocaine, but differ from cocaine mainly in that they have no abuse potential and do not act on the sympathoadrenergic system (i.e., do not produce hypertension or local vasoconstriction, except for ropivacaine and

---

T.M. Halaszynski, D.M.D., M.D., M.B.A. (✉)
Department of Anesthesiology, Yale University School of Medicine and Yale-New Haven Hospital, 333 Cedar Street, P.O. Box 208051, New Haven, CT 06520-8051, USA
e-mail: Thomas.Halaszynski@yale.edu

mepivacaine that may produce weak vasoconstriction). Local anesthetics vary in their pharmacological properties, and they are used in various techniques of local anesthesia such as topical anesthesia (surface), infiltration, and nerve or nerve plexus blockade.

Injectable local anesthetics are medicines given by injection to numb and provide pain relief to some part of the body during surgery and dental procedures. They are usually administered by a trained health care professional and in a doctor's office or hospital. Some commonly used injectable local anesthetics include procaine (Novocain), lidocaine (Dalcaine, Dilocaine, L-Caine, Nervocaine, Xylocaine, and other brands), bupivacaine (Marcaine), and tetracaine (Pontocaine). Topical anesthetics such as benzocaine, lidocaine, dibucaine, pramoxine, butamben, and tetracaine relieve pain and itching by anesthetizing the nerve endings in the skin and mucous membranes and are often applied prior to local anesthetic injection. These products are available as creams, ointments, sprays, lotions, and gels. Non-injectable dental anesthetics are intended for pain relief in the mouth or throat. They may be used to relieve discomfort from dentures, braces, bridgework, teething pain, painful canker sores, toothaches, or throat pain. Non-injectable dental anesthetics are available with a doctor's prescription, while other forms may be purchased without a prescription, including products such as Num-Zit, Orajel, Chloraseptic lozenges, and Xylocaine.

Mechanism of Action of Local Anesthetics

Local anesthesia administration is a technique that is intended and capable of rendering a part of the body insensitive to pain without affecting consciousness. Local anesthetics may be defined as a chemical compound capable of producing a loss of sensation in a circumscribed area of the body by reversible inhibition of neural conduction. Progressive increases in the concentrations of local anesthetics result in interruption of transmission of autonomic, sensory, and motor neural impulses and hence production of autonomic nervous system blockade, sensory anesthesia, and skeletal muscle paralysis in the areas innervated by the affected nerves. Local anesthesia will permit patients to undergo maxillofacial and dental procedures with reduced pain and distress. In many situations, local anesthesia can be safer and without many of the potential risks associated with GA and IV sedation (i.e., cardiovascular and respiratory depression). It can also be used for relief of nonsurgical pain and to enable diagnosis of the cause of certain chronic pain conditions.

Chemistry and classification identify local anesthetics as weak bases with pKa's>7.4 (except benzocaine, pKa 3.8). Local anesthetics consist of both a:

- Lipophilic aromatic group (benzene ring) and a
- Hydrophilic group (tertiary amine) connected together by an intermediate chain (Fig. 6.1)

The intermediate chain configuration is responsible for separating local anesthetic medications in one of the two groups—amide or ester type of local anesthetic drugs (Table 6.1). The chemical differences between the two groups of anesthetics

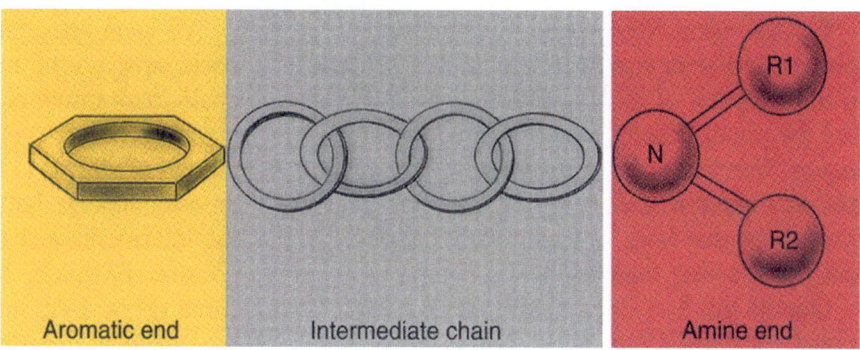

Fig. 6.1 Basic structure of local anesthetics

Table 6.1 Classification of local anesthetics (determined by type of intermediate chain)

Amino ester intermediate chain: Ester –COO– link	Amino amide intermediate chain: Amide –NH– link
• Cocaine	• Lidocaine
• Procaine	• Bupivacaine
• Chloroprocaine	• Mepivacaine
• Tetracaine	• Prilocaine
• Benzocaine	• Ropivacaine
Metabolism: Plasma by pseudo-cholinesterase	Metabolism: Enzymatic degradation in the liver (accumulation may occur in those with liver disease)

Esters have one "i" in drug name, while amides have two "i"s in the name

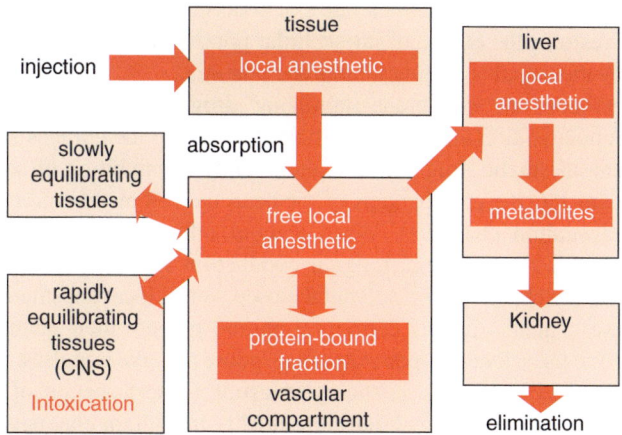

Fig. 6.2 Pharmacokinetics of injected local anesthetics

result from their mechanisms of metabolism. Esters are metabolized in the plasma by pseudo-cholinesterase, while amides undergo enzymatic degradation in the liver by aromatic hydroxylation (Fig. 6.2).

Table 6.2 Classification and physiologic characteristics of nerve fibers

Nerve fiber type	A-alpha	A-beta	A-gamma	A-delta	B	C
Function	Motor	Touch/pressure	Proprioception and motor tone	Pain/temperature	Preganglionic autonomic	Pain/temperature
Diameter (μm)	12–20	5–12	3–6	2–5	1–3	0.5–1.0
Conduction speed (m/s)	70–120	30–70	30–70	12–30	3–14	1.2

Reviewing the anatomy, physiology, and classification of nerve characteristics and nerve conduction (Table 6.2) is necessary before any discussion of local anesthetics, but basically, nerves transmit sensation(s) as a result of the propagation of electrical impulses. This propagation is accomplished by alternating the ion gradient across the nerve cell wall or axolemma. In the normal resting state, the nerve has a negative membrane potential (−70 mV), and this resting potential is determined by the concentration gradients of two major ions, Na^+ and K^+, and the relative membrane permeability to these ions. Then, when a nerve is stimulated, depolarization of the nerve occurs, and impulse propagation progresses. The entry of sodium ions causes the transmembrane electric potential to increase from the resting potential, and once the potential reaches a threshold level (approximately −55 mV), a rapid influx of sodium ions ensues. Sodium channels in the membrane become activated, and sodium ion permeability increases; the nerve membrane is depolarized (+35 mV). Once membrane depolarization is complete, the membrane becomes impermeable to sodium ions again, and the conductance of potassium ions into the cell increases. The process restores the excess of intracellular potassium and extracellular sodium and reinstates the negative resting membrane potential.

Local anesthetics are "membrane-stabilizing" drugs, and they reversibly decrease the rate of depolarization and repolarization of excitable membranes such as nociceptors. Local anesthetic drug action is due mainly to inhibition of sodium influx through sodium-specific ion channels of the neuronal cell membrane (the so-called voltage-gated sodium channels). When sodium influx is interrupted, an action potential cannot arise and neural signal conduction is inhibited. By selectively binding to sodium channels in inactivated closed states, local anesthetic molecules stabilize these channels in this configuration and prevent their change from the resting-closed to the activated-open states in response to nerve impulses. The receptor site is theorized to be located at the cytoplasmic (inner) portion of the sodium channel. Local anesthetic drugs bind more readily to sodium channels in the activated state; thus, onset of neuronal blockade is faster in neurons that are firing rapidly. This is often referred to as "state-dependent blockade."

All local anesthetics are considered weak bases and are often formulated as the hydrochloride salt to render them water soluble (Table 6.3). At the chemical's pKa, the protonated or ionized and unprotonated or unionized forms of local anesthetic

Table 6.3 Physical, chemical, and biological properties of common local anesthetics

Agent	Lipid solubility	Relative potency	pKa	Onset	Protein binding	Duration (min)
Low potency						
• Procaine	1	1	8.9	Slow	6	60–90
• Chloroprocaine	1	1	9.1	Fast	–	30–60
Intermediate potency						
• Mepivacaine	2	2	7.6	Fast	75	120–240
• Lidocaine	3.6	2	7.7	Fast	65	90–200
High potency						
• Tetracaine	80	8	8.6	Slow	80	180–600
• Bupivacaine	30	8	8.1	Intermediate	95	180–600

molecules exist in an equilibrium, but only the unionized anesthetic molecule diffuses readily across cell membranes. Once the anesthetic is inside the cell (diffusion through the cell membrane), the local anesthetic molecules will be in equilibrium, with the formation of the ionized form that will not readily pass back out of the cell. This is referred to as "ion trapping." In the protonated or the ionized form, the molecule binds to the local anesthetic binding site, near the cytoplasmic end, on the inside of the ion channel.

Nerve fibers are sensitive to local anesthetics, but generally, nerve fibers with a smaller diameter tend to be more sensitive than larger fibers. Myelinated nerve fibers tend to be more sensitive than non-myelinated fibers. Therefore, local anesthetics generally block nerve conduction in the following order: small myelinated axons (responsible for carrying nociceptive impulses), non-myelinated axons, and finally large myelinated axons. Hence, development of a differential block can often be observed (i.e., pain sensation is blocked more readily than other sensory modalities) as the effectiveness of the administered local anesthetic develops.

Techniques of Local Anesthetic Administration

There are several forms of orofacial anesthesia along with a host of various block techniques for procedures that are commonly performed for maxillofacial and dental interventions (Table 6.4). Mastery of this specialty, within dental anesthesiology, deals with the management of pain through the use of such varied techniques. Included in the armamentarium for dental anesthesia includes, but is not limited to, local anesthetic drugs and other anesthetics (nitrous oxide, eugenol, topical anesthetics, GA, opioids, IV sedation, etc), along with various techniques of nerve and nerve plexus blockade. Prior to practicing orofacial anesthesia techniques, an understanding of applied anatomy [1] is a prerequisite to maximize efficiency and reduce iatrogenic events.

There are various factors that may affect the pain of an intracutaneous local anesthetic injection. These include the preparation used, gauge of the needle stylus, area

Table 6.4 Types of orofacial/local anesthetic injections/nerve block techniques

Electrical nerve blocks	Technology involving electrical current to block generation/reception of pain signals
Branch block	Blocks reception of pain for one quadrant of the mouth (typically given in the buccal surface; example: IAB, MNB)
Dental block	Injected below the tooth in question (usually for minor procedures such as tooth fillings)
Palatal block	Injected into the hard palate, useful in numbing the maxillary teeth
Intraosseous	Injection directly into the osseous (bone) structure surrounding a tooth
Intrapulpal	Injection given directly into the pulp of the tooth to completely desensitize the tooth
Acupuncture or acupressure	An alternative to chemical (local anesthetics) or electrical blocks (rarely used)

IAB inferior alveolar nerve block, *MNB* mental nerve block

Table 6.5 Properties of some commonly used dental local anesthetics

Agent	Bupivacain	Lidocaine	Mepivacaine	Prilocaine
Molecular weight	288	234	246	220
pKa	8.1	7.7	7.8	7.7
Distribution coefficient	27.5	46.4	19.3	20.5
Protein binding rate	95 %	77 %	78 %	55 %
Relative potency	16	4	4	4
Relative toxicity	8	2	1.8	1.5
Ratio of potency:toxicity	2	2	2.2	2.7
Elimination half time	162 min	96 min	114 min	93 min
Max recommended dose (70 kg)[a]	90 mg	300–500 mg[b]	400–500 mg[b]	400–600 mg[b]

[a]With epinephrine
[b]Recommendations can vary

of the body injected, volume of solution used, speed of injection, temperature of the injected local anesthetic solution, and deep or superficial intracutaneous injection, along with the variable of individual patient characteristics.

Local anesthetics are capable of blocking almost every nerve between the peripheral nerve endings to the central nervous system. Table 6.5 identifies some of the commonly used local anesthetic drugs used for injection and infiltration modalities in orofacial procedure protocols. The most peripheral technique is topical anesthesia to the skin, oral cavity, and other body surface. Small and large peripheral nerves can be anesthetized individually (peripheral nerve block) or in anatomic nerve bundles (plexus anesthesia).

Injection of local anesthetics is often painful, but a number of methods can be used to decrease this pain including buffering of the solution with bicarbonate and warming of the drug prior to use [2].

There are several clinical techniques used for the administration of local anesthetics that include the following:

- *Surface anesthesia*—application of local anesthetic spray, solution, or cream to the skin or the mucous membrane. The effect is short lasting and is limited to the area of contact.

- *Infiltration anesthesia*—injection of local anesthetic into the tissue to be anesthetized. Surface and infiltration anesthesia are collectively topical anesthesia.
- *Field block*—subcutaneous injection of local anesthetic in an area bordering on the intended site to be anesthetized.
- *Peripheral nerve block*—injection of local anesthetic in the vicinity of a peripheral nerve to anesthetize that nerve's area of innervation.
- *Plexus anesthesia*—injection of local anesthetic in the vicinity of a nerve plexus, often inside a tissue compartment that limits the diffusion of the drug away from the intended site of action.

The anesthetic effect extends to the innervation areas of several or all nerves stemming from the plexus.

Dental Local Anesthetics

Dental treatment and oral maxillofacial procedures are generally performed under local anesthesia, which has reached a high level of efficacy and safety. However, there continues to remain some requirements for dental local anesthetics including:

1. A high intrinsic activity, which ensures complete anesthesia for dental treatment
2. A rapid onset
3. An adequate duration of anesthesia in the range from 30 to 60 min for standard dental treatment
4. A low systemic toxicity
5. A high efficacy–toxicity ratio
6. A low overall incidence of serious adverse effects

Most of the modern amide-type local anesthetics fulfill many of the above conditions very well. On principle, every local anesthetic can be used in dentistry. Nevertheless, a few substances are more frequently or regularly used for orofacial anesthesia including lidocaine and bupivacaine, the most commonly used substances. Other local anesthetics are also used in dentistry and maxillofacial procedures for special indications such as mepivacaine and prilocaine. Anesthetic preparations for dental use differ from those for nondental use. For example, the concentration of local anesthetics for dental use is often higher, because the volume is limited as to how much can be injected into the oral mucosa (e.g., palatal injection or periodontal ligament (PDL) injection).

Commercially prepared local anesthetic solutions may contain a vasoconstrictor agent, mostly epinephrine, in concentrations varying from 5 µg/ml (1:200,000) to 20 µg/ml (1:50,000). The rationale for combining a vasoconstrictor agent with local anesthetic drugs is to prolong the duration of action of the anesthetic agent and to decrease the rate of absorption (i.e., vasoconstriction of the surrounding vasculature) from the site of administration in order to reduce the potential systemic toxicity. Bupivacaine is typically utilized as a 0.5 % solution without vasoconstrictor, because the duration of the anesthetic effect may already last as long as 6 h. It should be noted that newer preparations (e.g., Exparel™), including a preparation with a liposomial injectable suspension, have demonstrable plasma levels of bupivacaine for up to 96 h. Lidocaine is available as a 2 or a 3 % solution with 1:50,000 to 1:100,000 epinephrine. Commercial preparations of mepivacaine are 2 % solutions with 1:66,666 to 1:100,000 epinephrine or without a vasoconstrictor. Prilocaine is available as a 3 % solution with felypressin as a vasoconstrictor. Local anesthetic solutions for injection within the oral cavity are usually supplied in single-dose cartridges most often containing 1.8 ml (1.7 ml injectable) (Table 6.5).

Techniques of Dental Local Anesthesia Administration

With local infiltration techniques, small nerve endings in the area of the dental treatment are flooded with local anesthetic solution, therefore preventing them from becoming stimulated and creating an impulse. The local infiltration technique is commonly used in anesthesia of the maxillary teeth as well as the mandibular incisors and most soft tissue procedures. Infiltration procedures can be performed in the maxilla due to the thin cortical nature of the bone, and it involves injecting tissues immediately around the surgical site (supraperiosteal, intraseptal, and PDL injections). These field blocks permit local anesthetic to be deposited near a larger terminal branch of a nerve.

In nerve block anesthesia (conduction anesthesia), the local anesthetic solution is deposited within close proximity to a main nerve trunk, thus preventing afferent impulses from traveling centrally beyond that point. Nerve block is used in anesthesia of the inferior alveolar (mandibular) nerve, lingual nerve, buccal nerve, greater palatine nerve, and nasopalatine nerve. Nerve block technique(s) is required for anesthesia of mandibular molars and premolars because anesthetic solution is usually not able to penetrate the compact vestibular bone of the mandible. Thus, local infiltration technique(s) does not provide a complete or a successful anesthesia. Nerve blocks consist of local anesthetic deposited near main nerve trunks usually distant from the operative site (posterior superior alveolar, infraorbital, middle superior alveolar, and anterior superior alveolar nerves).

The posterior superior alveolar nerve block is used to anesthetize the pulpal tissue, corresponding alveolar bone, and buccal gingival tissue to the maxillary first, second, and third molars. The technique consists of identifying the area of insertion (height of mucobuccal fold between first and second molars) and then angling at 45° superiorly and medially. No resistance should be felt; if bony contact is made, then angle is too medial and reposition laterally is required; then insert about 15–20 mm, and inject the local anesthetic subsequent to confirmation of negative aspiration.

The middle superior alveolar nerve block is used to anesthetize the maxillary premolars, corresponding alveolus, and buccal gingival tissue. It is present in about 28 % of the population and used if the infraorbital block fails to anesthetize the premolars. The technique involved identifies the height of the mucobuccal fold (area of insertion) in the area of first/second premolars and inserts to a depth of about 10–15 mm followed by injection of around 0.9–1.2 cc of local.

The anterior superior alveolar nerve block is used to anesthetize the maxillary canine, lateral incisor, central incisor, alveolus, and buccal gingival. The technique identifies the area of insertion (height of mucobuccal fold in area of lateral incisor and canine) and then inserts the block needle around 10–15 mm followed by injecting 0.9–1.2 cc of local.

An infraorbital nerve block is used to anesthetize the maxillary first and second premolars, canine, lateral incisor, central incisor, corresponding alveolar bone, and buccal gingival (it combines both the anterior and middle superior alveolar nerve blocks), in addition to anesthesia of the lower eyelid, lateral aspect of nasal skin tissue, and skin of infraorbital region. The technique involves palpation of the infraorbital foramen by extraorally placing a thumb or an index finger in the region and then retracting the upper lip and buccal mucosa (area of insertion is the mucobuccal fold of the first premolar/canine area). Subsequent to contacting bone in the infraorbital region, inject 0.9–1.2 cc of local anesthetic.

The greater palatine nerve block can be used to anesthetize the palatal soft tissue of the teeth posterior to the maxillary canine and corresponding alveolus and hard palate. The technique finds the area of insertion at ~1 cm medial from first/second maxillary molars on the hard palate and then palpates with needle to find the greater palatine foramen (depth is usually less than 10 mm). Subsequently, utilize pressure with an elevator or a mirror handle to desensitize the region at the time of injection of 0.3–0.5 cc of local anesthetic.

The nasopalatine block can be used to anesthetize the soft and hard tissue of the maxillary anterior palate from canine to canine. The technique involves locating the site of injection (incisive papilla into incisive foramen) to a depth of penetration of less than 10 mm followed by injecting 0.3–0.5 cc of local anesthetic (pressure over area at the time of injection can be used to decrease injection pain).

The maxillary nerve block (V2 block) is used to anesthetize maxillary teeth, alveolus, hard and soft tissue on the palate, gingiva, skin of the lower eyelid, and lateral aspect of nose, cheek, upper lip skin, and mucosa on the side blocked. Two techniques exist for blockade of V2—high tuberosity approach and the greater palatine canal approach. High tuberosity approach technique finds area of injection at the height of mucobuccal fold of the maxillary second molar and needle advanced at 45° superior and medial (same as in the posterior alveolar nerve block). The needle is inserted ~30 mm followed by injecting ~1.8 cc of local anesthetic. Greater palatine canal technique uses insertion of the greater palatine canal as the target area of the maxillary nerve in the pterygopalatine fossa. First, perform a greater palatine block, wait for 3–5 min, then insert needle in previous area, walk into greater palatine foramen, and insert to depth of ~30 mm followed by injection of 1.8 cc of local anesthetic solution.

Infiltration techniques do not work well in the adult mandible due to the dense cortical bone. Therefore, nerve blocks are used to anesthetize the inferior alveolar, lingual, and buccal nerves that provide anesthesia to the pulpal, alveolar, lingual, and buccal gingival tissue; skin of lower lip; and medial aspect of chin on the side injected. The technique involves blocking the inferior alveolar nerve prior to entry into the mandibular lingula on the medial aspect of the mandibular ramus. A few techniques can be used for this nerve block including an inferior alveolar nerve block and an Akinosi closed-mouth mandibular block. The technique of an inferior alveolar nerve block aims for needle insertion on the mucous membrane on the medial border of the mandibular ramus at the intersection of a horizontal line and vertical line (anteroposterior plane). Location of needle insertion is at a height of 6–10 mm above the occlusal table of the mandibular teeth in an anteroposterior plane just lateral to the pterygomandibular raphe. The depth of insertion is about 25 mm, and the approach area of injection is from the contralateral premolar region using the non-dominant hand to retract the buccal soft tissue (thumb in coronoid notch of mandible and index finger on posterior border of extraoral mandible). Then inject ~0.5–1.0 cc of local anesthetic, and continue to inject ~0.5 cc of local on removal from the injection site to anesthetize the branch of the lingual nerve. Inject additional anesthetic solution into the coronoid notch region of the mandible in the mucous membrane distal and buccal to most distal molar to perform a long buccal nerve block. An Akinosi closed-mouth mandibular block is a useful technique for infected patients with trismus, fractured mandibles, mentally handicapped individuals, and children. It provides same areas of anesthesia as the inferior alveolar nerve block. The area of insertion is the soft tissue overlying the medial border of the mandibular ramus directly adjacent to the maxillary tuberosity. Insert the needle to a depth of 25 mm, and inject ~1.0–1.5 cc of local anesthetic followed by injecting additional anesthetic in the area of the long buccal nerve.

Terminal branches of the inferior alveolar nerve are mental and incisive nerves that provide sensory input for the lower lip skin, mucous membrane, and pulpal and alveolar tissue for the premolars, canine, and incisors on the side blocked. The area of injection for a mental nerve block is the mucobuccal fold at or anterior to the mental foramen that lies between the mandibular premolars. Depth of injection is ~5–6 mm; inject 0.5–1.0 cc of local anesthesia, and then message local anesthesia into tissue to manipulate into mental foramen in order to anesthetize the incisive branch.

In the PDL technique (intraligamentary injection), the local anesthetic solution is injected into the desmodontal space. The PDL technique is useful for anesthesia of mandibular molars and can be used as an alternative to the nerve block technique. Careful PDL injection is often painless, and the anesthetic effect is limited to the pulp and desmodontal nerve of the tooth anesthetized. Duration of anesthesia is in the range of 15–20 min, which allows for most routine dental treatments. The PDL injection is useful for extremely anxious patients and children, who do not tolerate conventional local anesthetic administration techniques. For a PDL technique, a high concentration of the local anesthetic is required due to the limited volume used, which can be injected into the narrow desmodontal space. The dose of anesthetic solution for a PDL injection, which is required for complete anesthesia, is lower than in an infiltration or a nerve block technique.

Local anesthesia techniques used in oral and maxillofacial surgery procedures are based on proper understanding and overview of anatomy of maxillary and mandibular nervous system innervation including, but not limited to, anatomical consideration of the trigeminal nerve (Table 6.6). Anatomical considerations for the

Table 6.6 Anatomical consideration of the trigeminal nerve

Sensory divisions	Motor divisions
• Ophthalmic division V1 • Maxillary division V2 • Mandibular division V3	• Masticatory-masseter, temporalis, medial, and lateral pterygoids • Mylohyoid • Anterior belly of the digastric • Tensor tympani • Tensor veli palatini

host of nerve branches and anatomical locations of nerves within their distribution, communication, and termination must first be understood. In addition, instrumentation for performing such techniques must be understood and is available such as anesthetic carpules, syringe types (aspirating and non-aspirating), needles (assortment of multiple gauges and lengths), mouth props, and retractors.

Undesired Effects from Local Anesthetic Administration

Whenever local anesthesia is being used, it should always be remembered that both anatomical and pharmacological considerations could result in complications, ranging from temporary discomfort for the patient to the rare event of patient death [3]. While generally safe, local anesthetic agents can be toxic if used in excessive doses or administered improperly. Even when administered properly, patients may still experience unintended reactions to local anesthetic agents [4]. Excessive doses of local anesthetic drugs may be unintentionally administered in several ways such as the following: (1) Repetitive (small) doses of local anesthetic to achieve an adequate level of anesthesia (may lead to eventual administration of toxic doses); (2) injection of anesthesia in a confined space may result in excessive fluid pressure (this may damage nerves); and (3) doses intended for intra-support-tissue administration may be accidentally delivered as intravascular injection, resulting in accelerated systematic absorption. The toxic effects of local anesthetics can be classified as either localized or systemic adverse effects or both.

Localized Adverse Effects from Local Anesthetic Drugs

Dentists and oral surgeons administer thousands of local anesthetic injections every day with few reports of serious complications [5]. However, misjudging the anatomy involved during local anesthetic administration may result in inadequate or incomplete anesthesia, but also in other complications such as paresthesia, bleeding, or hematoma formation or in serious systemic complications. Anatomical considerations should be kept in mind when administering local anesthetic medications. In particular, attention provided toward safety mechanisms that may minimize the risk of nerve or vascular injury as well as systemic complications; in addition, consideration of local anesthetics and needle placement with regard to location of nerves, blood vessels, and glands along with a review of injection protocols that can minimize associated risks.

Until the influences from local anesthetic administration have subsided ("wear off"), patients should be instructed how to maintain care so as not to inadvertently injure the anesthetized area. When the anesthetics are used in the mouth, patients should be instructed not to eat or chew gum until "normal" sensations and feeling return. Side effects of regional or local anesthetics vary depending on the type of anesthetic used and the mechanism of administration. Any unusual symptoms following the use of local anesthesia administration requires immediate attention.

A cause of local toxicity is allergic reaction to para-aminobenzoic acid (PABA), and these reactions range from urticaria to anaphylaxis. PABA is a metabolic product of the degradation of the ester class of local anesthetics, such as procaine (Novocain), benzocaine, and, to a lesser degree, the amide class anesthetics such as lidocaine and prilocaine. PABA is also a metabolic by-product of methylparaben, used as a preservative in multi-dose vials of lidocaine. When an allergic response to an injected anesthetic does occur, it is most likely due to the ester class local anesthetics. The amide class of local anesthetics is far less likely to produce allergic reaction [6].

Risks Associated with Needle Placement Techniques

When used properly, local anesthetics are safe and have few major side effects. Some potential disadvantages of nerve block techniques include an increased risk of trauma to the nerve fiber as well as an accidental intravasculr or intraneural injection of the local anesthetic solution. The risk of temporary or permanent nerve damage varies between different locations along an individual nerve fiber and type of nerve block being performed [7]. However, in high doses, local anesthetics may have toxic effects caused by being absorbed through the bloodstream into the rest of the body (systemic toxicity). The result of such an occurrence may significantly affect a patient's breathing, heartbeat, blood pressure, and other body functions. Therefore, because of these potential toxic effects, equipment for emergency care should be available in areas where local anesthetics are being administered.

Recovery and Causes from Local Anesthetic Localized Adverse Effects

The local adverse effects of anesthetic agents include neurovascular manifestations such as prolonged anesthesia (numbness) and paresthesia (tingling, feeling of "pins and needles," or strange sensations). These are usually symptoms indicative of localized nerve impairment or nerve branch damage [8]. Permanent nerve damage after a peripheral nerve block is rare. Symptoms are very likely to resolve within a few weeks. The vast majority of patients affected (92–97 %) will recover within 4–6 weeks. 99 % of these people usually recovered completely within a year [9]. It is estimated that between 1 in 5,000 and 1 in 30,000 nerve blocks result in some degree of permanent persistent nerve damage [10]. It has been further suggested that adverse symptoms from nerve damage may continue to improve for up to 18 months following the initial injury.

Causes of localized untoward neurologic symptoms from local anesthetic administration include: (1) neurotoxicity due to an allergenic reaction, (2) potential for excessive fluid pressure due to injection in a confined space, (3) severing of nerve fibers or support tissue with the needle, (4) an injection-site hematoma that may put pressure on a nerve or a nerve fiber, and/or (5) injection-site infection that produces inflammatory pressure on the nerve and/or necrosis.

Systemic Adverse Effects from Local Anesthetic Medications

General systemic adverse affects may be due to the pharmacological effects of the particular anesthetic agent used. The conduction of electric impulses follows a similar mechanism in peripheral nerves, the central nervous system, and the heart. The effects of local anesthetics are therefore not specific for the signal conduction in peripheral nerves. Side effects on the central nervous system and the heart may be severe and potentially fatal with inadvertent intravenous administration of a large bolus of local anesthetic solution. However, toxicity usually occurs only at plasma levels that are rarely reached if proper anesthetic techniques and administration protocols are adhered to properly. In addition, patients may exhibit varying degrees of allergenic reactions to the anesthetic compounds.

Hypersensitivity/Allergy to Local Anesthetics

Adverse reactions to local anesthetics (especially the esters) are not uncommon, but true allergy is very rare. Non-allergic reactions may resemble an allergy due to similar manifestations. Serious allergic reactions to local anesthetic medications are rare and usually attributable to factors other than the anesthetic (i.e., inadvertent intravascular injection). Allergic reactions to the ester local anesthetics are more commonly due to a sensitivity of the local anesthetic drug metabolite produced, PABA, and do not result in cross-allergy to the amide class of locals. Therefore, amides can be used as alternatives in those patients with adverse or allergic reactions to the ester local anesthetics. In some cases, skin tests and provocative challenge may be necessary to establish a diagnosis of true allergy to either class of local anesthetic. There are also cases of allergy to paraben derivatives, which are often added as preservatives to local anesthetic solutions.

Central Nervous System

Under certain circumstances and depending on local tissue concentrations of local anesthetics, there may be excitatory or depressant effects on the central nervous system.

At lower concentrations, a relatively selective depression of inhibitory neurons results in cerebral excitation, which in the extreme may lead to generalized convulsions. A profound depression of brain functions occurs at higher concentrations that may lead to coma, respiratory arrest, and death. Such tissue concentrations are usually due to very high plasma levels after accidental IV injection of a large dose of local anesthetic drug. Another possibility is the rare event of direct exposure to the central nervous system through the cerebral spinal fluid caused by aberrant needle tip placement and accidental injection into the subarachnoid space.

Cardiovascular System

The conductive system of the heart is quite sensitive to the action of local anesthetics, although less so than the central nervous system. Systemic toxic reactions to administered local anesthetics become progressive as the level of the anesthetic agent in the blood rises. The initial symptoms usually suggest some form of central nervous system excitation (i.e., ringing in the ears [tinnitus], a metallic taste in the mouth, or tingling or numbness of the mouth), but advanced symptoms may include motor twitching in the periphery followed by grand mal seizures, coma, and eventually respiratory arrest. At higher local anesthetic concentration levels, cardiac arrhythmias, hypotension, and cardiovascular collapse may occur [11]. Cardiovascular effects are primarily those of direct myocardial depression and bradycardia, which may lead to cardiovascular collapse.

Treatment of Local Anesthetic Overdose: "Lipid Rescue"

There is evidence that intralipid, a commonly available IV lipid emulsion, can be effective in treating severe cardiotoxicity secondary to local anesthetic overdose ("lipid rescue") [12]. Lipid rescue administration should be considered and may be indicated due to inadvertent intravascular injection of a large bolus(s) of local anesthetic medications that results in asystole or cardiovascular collapse [13].

Acknowledgement None declared.

Conflict of Interest None declared.

References

1. Netter F. Atlas of human anatomy. CIBA. 1989
2. Colaric KB, Overton DT, Moore K. Pain reduction in lidocaine administration through buffering and warming. Am J Emerg Med. 1998;16(4):353–6.
3. Hersh EV, Helpin ML, Evans OB. Local anesthetic mortality: report of a case. ASDC J Dent Child. 1991;58:489–91.

4. Mather LE. The acute toxicity of local anesthetics. Drug Metab Toxicol. 2010;6(11): 1313–32.
5. Malamed SF. Handbook of local anesthesia. 4th ed. St. Louis: Mosby; 1997. p. 143–259.
6. Fuzier R, Lapeyre-Mestre M, Mertes PM, et al. Immediate—and delayed-type allergic reactions to amide local anesthetics: clinical features and skin testing. Pharmacoepidemiol Drug Saf. 2009;18(7):595–601.
7. Haas DA. Articaine and paresthesia: epidemiological studies. J Am Coll Dent. 2006;73(3): 5–10.
8. Haas DA, Lennon D. A 21-year retrospective study of reports of paresthesia following local anesthetic administration. J Can Dent Assoc. 1995;61(4):319–20. 323–6, 329–30.
9. Garisto GA, Gaffen AS, Lawrence HP, et al. Occurrence of paresthesia after dental local anesthetic administration in the United States. J Am Dent Assoc. 2010;141(7):836–44.
10. Pogrel MA. Permanent nerve damage from inferior alveolar nerve blocks—an update to include articaine. J Calif Dent Assoc. 2007;35(4):271–3.
11. Corcoran W, Butterworth J, Weller RS, et al. Local anesthetic—induced cardiac toxicity: a survey of contemporary practice strategies among academic anesthesiology departments. Anesth Analg. 2006;103(5):13226.
12. Weinberg GL, VadeBoncouer T, Ramaraju GA, et al. Pretreatment or resuscitation with a lipid infusion shifts the dose-response to bupivacaine-induced asystole in rats. Anesthesiology. 1998;88:1071–5.
13. Picard J, Meek T. Lipid emulsion to treat overdose of local anesthetic: the gift of the glob. Anesthesia. 2006;61:107–9.

Chapter 7
Analgesics and Adjuvants for the Management of Orofacial Pain Across Age Groups

Ian Laughlin and Anita H. Hickey

Introduction

The orofacial region is critical for survival due to its role in eating and drinking, identity and self-esteem, and communication and expressions of love and emotional connection. Orofacial pain is comparatively less tolerated than pain in other body areas due to its disproportionate representation in the cerebral cortex somatosensory homunculus. The individual with severe orofacial pain can therefore be at significant risk of deficient nutritional intake, dehydration, and withdrawal from essential social interactions.

Pain, chiefly chronic pain, is a multidimensional experience, with sensory-discriminative, emotional, cultural, and cognitive components. It is influenced by environmental, hormonal, and mood fluctuations; neurologic and inflammatory changes; as well as cognitive and physiologic memory of previous encounters with pain. The successful treatment of pain requires thorough assessment of the cause and character of the pain, its underlying pathophysiology, and contribution of psychological, social, spiritual, and practical issues. Successful management must include not only pharmacologic interventions but also adequate follow-up with verbal and written education of the patient, family, and caregivers to assure compliance and decrease the incidence of adverse effects and outcomes of medications. Based on the complexity and chronicity of pain, its management may also require important interdisciplinary team members including nursing, social workers, pharmacists, chaplains, physiotherapists, occupational therapists, and stage of life specialists. Integration of cognitive behavioral therapies, physical medicine, and rehabilitation approaches, together with evidence-based alternative and mind–body approaches, improves patient satisfaction and well-being, decreases pain medication requirements, and lessens side effects compared to the use of medications alone [1].

I. Laughlin, M.D. • A.H. Hickey, M.D. (✉)
Naval Medical Center, San Diego, CA, USA
e-mail: Anita.Hickey@med.navy.mil

Elucidating the qualities and characteristics of orofacial pain disorders and syndromes is essential for successful selection of therapies, according to various levels of evidence and based on rigorous research-based classification and diagnostic criteria [2, 3].

In addition to providing a concise and complete resource for dosing of the various classes and of pain medications and adjunctive medications in the treatment of orofacial pain across the age range from neonates to geriatric patients, this chapter addresses the unique physiology of each age group as well as important alterations in pharmacokinetics which can occur at various ages and with common comorbidities as well as the importance of synergistic multimodal polypharmacy/analgesia [4].

Although this chapter focuses on the successful pharmacologic treatment of acute and chronic orofacial pain, it also highlights recent evidence, which allows us to decrease the risks associated with the development of chronic persistent pain in those individuals who are most susceptible [5–10].

The WHO Analgesic Ladder

The World Health Organization (WHO) developed a three-step approach in 1986 intended to act as a template for cancer pain management. By consensus, it has become a simple, validated method for sensible and judicious choice, delivery, and titration of various pain medication classes and formulations in acute and chronic benign pain in addition to pain associated with cancer and severe illness in all age groups.

WHO Ladder Step 1: Analgesics for Mild Pain

Acetaminophen

Both acetaminophen and nonsteroidal anti-inflammatory drugs (NSAIDs) act by inhibiting prostaglandin synthesis; however, acetaminophen does not inhibit platelets and has little anti-inflammatory activity. Acetaminophen is a common ingredient in many over-the-counter cold and flu remedies and is indicated for mild aches and pains and to reduce fever. It is metabolized by the liver P450 system with a toxic intermediate metabolite N-acetyl-p-benzoquinone imine (NAPQI), a topoisomerase poison which is very reactive and toxic to liver cells.

In recommended doses and in individuals with normal liver function, NAPQI is converted to a harmless metabolite by the antioxidant glutathione. Large doses of acetaminophen or preexisting impairment of liver function result in a reduced supply of glutathione, leading to potentially fatal hepatic centrilobular necrosis, and renal insufficiency; 4 g/day of acetaminophen in divided doses is reported as safe for patients aged 12 or greater in the absence of renal or hepatic or excess alcohol use. A maximum of 2.5 g/day are recommended for patients less than 50 kg. Individuals who drink greater than 60 g/day of alcohol or have a history of binge drinking should take a maximum of 2 g/day of acetaminophen. Toxicity at normally prescribed doses has been reported in dehydrated patients [11–15].

Nonsteroidal Anti-inflammatory Drugs

NSAIDs inhibit prostaglandin synthesis by acting at the cyclo-oxygenase family of enzymes. They have been found to have opioid-sparing effects and decrease opioid-related nausea and vomiting but not pruritus or urinary retention. NSAID use, in particular those with selective COX-1-inhibiting effects, is associated with an increased risk of myocardial infarction, stroke, and serious gastrointestinal events such as bleeding, ulceration, and perforation. Elderly patients, those with impaired renal function, heart failure, impaired hepatic function, and taking diuretics and angiotensin-converting enzymes (ACE) inhibitors are at significant risk of acute renal failure due to renal papillary necrosis. Upon immediate discontinuation of NSAID therapy recovery usually occurs [16].

WHO Step Ladder 2: Analgesics for Moderate Pain

The majority of short-acting oral opioids are formulated as fixed-dose combinations with nonopioid analgesics. The synergy of the opioid and nonopioid component has the advantage of an opioid-sparing effect and is also associated with decreased opioid-related nausea and vomiting. Their efficacy is limited, however, by the maximal safe dose for the acetaminophen, aspirin, or NSAID component. Physicians should be aware of the dose of adjuvant associated with each dosage form of opioid in order to prevent toxicity. In cases where the patient requires a greater dose of opioid than allowed by the combination drug, a pure opioid should be prescribed. The patient can still benefit from the adjuvant by supplementing the opioid with acetaminophen or NSAIDs at appropriate doses at regular intervals. Physicians and allied health providers who prescribe these medications should be aware that NSAID toxicity has been reported at standard doses in patients with impaired renal function and with greater than moderate chronic alcohol use and in malnourished or dehydrated children.

WHO Ladder Step 3: Severe Pain

Opioids are recognized as the most effective treatment for moderate to severe acute pain and cancer pain. The decision to administer opioids in chronic benign pain is controversial. In the setting of acute pain and cancer pain, reliable establishment of profound analgesia with dose escalation and a predicable dose-dependent response and lack of ceiling effects are seen. In chronic benign pain, opioid use is associated with tolerance and less predictable dose-dependent analgesic response. Opioid use is not associated with organ toxicity with the exception of methadone and toxic metabolites of meperidine, morphine, and propoxyphene. There is evidence that opioids can significantly reduce pain and improve mood and function in chronic nonmalignant pain including neuropathic, nociceptive, and mixed pain [17, 18]. Long-term efficacy of opioid use in the setting of chronic benign pain and risks associated with this application are not well established as no quality long-term studies of greater than 16 weeks have been performed [19, 20].

μ-Opioid agonists are the primary agents of choice in the acute pain setting with dose escalation associated with predicable side effects that increase in a dose-dependent fashion. Side effects may differ according to the opioid administered due to mediation of both analgesia and adverse side effects by the μ-opioid receptor. Care must be taken when patients are taking other medications with sedative or central nervous system depressant effects as these may be synergistic with the opioid resulting in greater than expected sedation and respiratory depression.

Opioids not only are more useful in chronic pain and neuropathic pain and have analgesic effects at the μ-opioid receptor but also act as N-methyl-D-aspartate (NMDA) receptor antagonists and have central neuromodulating effects through inhibition of reuptake of serotonin and norepinephrine, similar to many antidepressants.

Some opioids have all three properties (e.g., methadone). Opioids with agonist/antagonist properties such as buprenorphine have also been shown to be useful in chronic pain, in particular in elderly patients [20].

Addiction of patients to prescription opioids is reported to vary between 0.05 and 32 %, according to factors such as the medical setting, patient population served, and presence of risk factors such as a history of addiction or drug abuse, preadolescent sexual abuse, and major psychiatric conditions. Guidelines and screening tools have been established to increase the safety and efficacy of long-term opioid use [21–25].

Special Considerations for Pediatric, Obstetrical, and Elderly Patients

Pain Formulary Considerations in the Pediatric Patient Population

Considerable recent laboratory and clinical research has reported that long-term behavioral and personality changes may result from inadequate treatment of acute pain episodes in early life. Chronic pain is common in children and if inadequately treated leads to physical and emotional disability in adult life. A multidisciplinary approach to chronic pain in this population utilizing health psychology, pain management specialists, and physical rehabilitation is indicated when medication or pain management approaches alone are not successful [26–33].

Pain Formulary Considerations for the Pregnant Female Patient

In addition to consideration of the FDA classifications for administration of drugs during pregnancy, and WHO analgesic ladder guidelines, experts recommend administration of short-acting opioids if possible during pregnancy and nursing. For opioid-dependent pregnant females, consultation with a perinatologist and neonatologist should be obtained. Titration of long-acting opioids during pregnancy has been associated with poor fetal outcome including intrauterine death [34, 35].

If opioids are required by nursing mothers, short-acting opioids are recommended. There is little risk of transfer of opioid to the infant immediately after birth to approximately 4 days following delivery since milk production is minimal during this period. Since peak milk production occurs immediately after nursing, medication should be taken after nursing so that peak serum level of 1½ to 2 h does not coincide with peak milk production. Nursing is not recommended during the first 1–2 h after taking short-acting opioids. Current FDA labels for hydrocodone and oxycodone recommend against their use while nursing due to risk of sedation and withdrawal in the infant. Expert consensus and available evidence site infant sedation and opiate withdrawal in doses greater than 30–40 mg/day and recommend "pumping and dumping" to maintain breast milk during dosing above 30–40 mg/day and resuming when below this dose or when short-acting opioids have been discontinued.

Pharmacologic Management of Orofacial Pain in the Elderly

Expeditious control of orofacial pain is particularly important in the elderly patient. Orofacial pain may precipitate a decline in hydration or nutrition leading to a precipitous decline in health. Other functions essential for survival such as verbal communication and social skills may also be eroded. The need to rapidly intervene must be balanced with the significant risk of adverse events, side effects in this age group due to differences in absorption and excretion compared to younger patients, decline in organ systems in patients with multiple comorbidities, and increased risk of drug–drug interactions in patients taking multiple medications.

According to the American Geriatrics Society (AGS) guidelines, acetaminophen should be considered for the initial and ongoing treatment of persistent pain. COX 2 selective and nonselective COX inhibitor NSAIDs should be used only rarely in highly selected cases in this population due to increased risk of acute renal impairment, gastrointestinal bleeding, hypertension, and cardiovascular and cerebrovascular complications.

When acetaminophen is ineffective, the WHO ladder should be considered. When opioids are required, low doses of adjuvant analgesics may decrease the patient's opioid requirement. Other routes such as topical analgesics with limited systemic side effects should also be considered.

Renal impairment is an important consideration when opioids with active metabolites are considered as these are 90–95 % renally excreted. Morphine-3-glucuronide and morphine-6-glucuronide are two principal metabolites of morphine whose half-lives are longer than the parent drug. Dehydration, acute or chronic renal failure, and urinary tract infections are processes which impair renal clearance necessitating increases in the dosing intervals or decreases in dose. Decreased hepatic function may also require a decrease in opioid dose or an increase in the dosing interval.

Side effects such as sedation may require modification of dosing or trials of alternative opioids or routes. Excess sedation may also be due to too rapid escalation of dose or interaction with other CNS depressants. Psychostimulants may be helpful in alleviating mild sedation. Prompt treatment of constipation is essential due to persistence of this side effect even with chronic opioid use.

Application of nonpharmacologic modalities known to decrease opioid requirements such as cognitive approaches is an important means of reducing anxiety which is an independent risk factor for the development of chronic postoperative pain. Other research has demonstrated a 50 % reduction in the need for postoperative analgesics following the preoperative communication of compassion and concern by the surgeon or the anesthesiologist.

Acknowledgement None declared.

Conflict of Interest None declared.

References

1. Maizes V, et al. Integrative medicine and patient centered care. Explore (NY). 2009;5(5):277–89.
2. Oelesen J et al. Headache Classification Subcommittee of the International Headache Society. The International Classification of Headache Disorders 2nd Edn. Cephalgia 2004;24(1):8–152
3. de Leeuw R, The American Academy of Orofacial Pain, et al. Orofacial pain: guidelines for assessment, diagnosis, and management. 4th ed. Chicago: Quintessence Publishing Company, Inc.; 2008.
4. Elvir-Lazo OL. Postoperative pain management after ambulatory surgery: role of multimodal analgesia. Anesthesiol Clinc. 2010;28(2):217–24.
5. MacGregor AJ. The heritability of pain in humans. In: Mogil JS, editor. The genetics of pain, Progress in pain research and management, vol. 28. Seattle: IASP Press; 2004. p. 151–70.
6. Ophoff RA, Terwindt GM, Vergouwe MN, et al. Familial hemiplegic migraine and episodic ataxia type-2 are caused by mutations in the Ca2+ channel gene CACNL1A4. Cell. 1996;87:543–52.
7. Kusumi M, Araki H, Ijiri T, et al. Serotonin 2C receptor gene Cys23Ser polymorphism: a candidate genetic risk factor of migraine with aura in Japanese population. Acta Neurol Scand. 2004;109:407–9.
8. Estevez M, Gardner KL. Update on the genetics of migraine. Hum Genet. 2004;114:225–35.
9. Violon A, Giugea D. Familial models for chronic pain. Pain. 1984;18:199–203.
10. Edwards PW, Zeichner A, Kuczmierczyk AR, Boczkowski J. Familial pain models: the relationship between family history of pain and current pain experience. Pain. 1985;21:379–84.
11. Chun LJ, Tong MJ, Busuttil R, Hiatt JR. Acetaminophen hepatotoxicity and acute liver failure. J Clin Gastroenterol. 2009;43(4):342–9.

12. Amar PJ, Schiff ER. Acetaminophen safety and hepatotoxicity—where do we go from here? Expert Opin Drug Saf. 2007;6(4):341–55.
13. Zimmerman HJ, Maddrey WC. Acetaminophen (paracetamol) hepatotoxicity with regular intake of alcohol: analysis of instances of therapeutic misadventure. Hepatology. 1995;22(3):767–73.
14. Mehta S. Pediatric Gastroenterology, Postgraduate Institute of Medical Education and Research, Chandigarh, India Malnutrition and drugs: clinical implications. Dev Pharmacol Ther. 1990;15(3–4):159–65.
15. Mazer M, Perrone J. Acetaminophen-induced nephrotoxicity: pathophysiology, clinical manifestations, and management. J Med Toxicol. 2008;4(1):2–6.
16. Scanzello CR, Moskowitz NK, Gibofsky JD. The post-NSAID era: what to use now for the pharmacologic treatment of pain and inflammation in osteoarthritis. Curr Pain Headache Rep. 2007;11:415–22.
17. Furlan AD, Sandoval JA, Mailis-Gagnon A, Tunks E. Opioids for chronic noncancer pain: a meta-analysis of effectiveness and side effects. CMAJ. 2006;174:1589–94.
18. Kalso E, Allan L, Dellemijn PL, Faura CC, Ilias WK, Jensen TS, et al. Recommendations for using opioids in chronic non-cancer pain. Eur J Pain. 2003;7:381–6.
19. Kroenke K, Dregs EE, et al. Pharmacotherapy of chronic pain: a synthesis of recommendations from systematic reviews. Gen Hosp Psychiat. 2009;31:206–19.
20. Gallagher RM, Rosenthal LJ. Chronic pain and opiates: balancing pain control and risks in long-term opioid treatment. Arch Phys Med Rehabil. 2008;89(3 Suppl 1):S77–82.
21. Vadivelu N, Hines RL. Management of chronic pain in the elderly: focus on transdermal buprenorphine. Clin Interv Aging. 2008;3(3):421–30.
22. Kirsh KL, Fishman SM. Multimodal approaches to optimize outcomes of chronic opioid therapy in the management of chronic pain. Pain Med. 2011;S1:S1–11.
23. McCleane GJ. Intravenous infusion of phenytoin relieves neuropathic pain: a randomized, double-blinded, placebo-controlled, crossover study. Anesth Analg. 1999;89:985–8.
24. Lin TF, Yeh YC, et al. Effect of combining dexmedetomidine and morphine for intravenous patient-controlled analgesia. Br J Anesth. 2009;102(1):117–22.
25. Sigtermans MJ, et al. Ketamine produces effective and long-term pain relief in patients with complex regional pain syndrome type 1. Pain. 2009;145:304–11.
26. Anand KJ. Pain, plasticity, and premature birth: a prescription for permanent suffering? Nat Med. 2000;6:971–3.
27. Grunau RE. Long-term consequences of pain in human neonates. In: Anand KJS, Stevens BJ, McGrath PJ, editors. Pain in neonates. 2nd ed. New York, NY: Elsevier; 2000. p. 55–76.
28. Taddio A, Katz J, Ilersich AL, Koren G. Effect of neonatal circumcision on pain response during subsequent routine vaccination. Lancet. 1997;349:599–603.
29. Reynolds ML, Fitzgerald M. Long-term sensory hyperinnervation following neonatal skin wounds. J Comp Neurol. 1995;358:487–98.
30. Ruda MA, Ling QD, Hohmann AG, Peng YB, Tachibana T. Altered nociceptive neuronal circuits after neonatal peripheral inflammation. Science. 2000;289:628–31.
31. Perquin CW, Hazebroek-Kampschreur AA, Hunfeld JA, van Suijlekom SLW, Passchier J, van der Wouden JC. Chronic pain among children and adolescents: physician consultation and medication use. Clin J Pain. 2000;16:229–35.
32. Campo JV, Di LC, Chiappetta L, et al. Adult outcomes of pediatric recurrent abdominal pain: do they just grow out of it? Pediatrics. 2001;108:E1.
33. Lee BH, Scharff L, Sethna NF, et al. Physical therapy and cognitive-behavioral treatment for complex regional pain syndromes. J Pediatr. 2002;141:135–40.
34. Jones HE, Martin PR, Heil SH. Treatment of opioid dependent pregnant women: clinical and research issues. J Subst Abuse Treat. 2008;35(3):245–59.
35. Kandall SR, Albin S, et al. The narcotic-dependent mother: fetal and neonatal consequences. Early Hum Dev. 1977;1(2):159–69.

Chapter 8
Cognitive Behavioral Therapy in Pain Management

Thomas M. Halaszynski

Introduction

> It's not things that trouble us but the views we take of them.
>
> —Epictetus

Pain is notoriously difficult to treat, and although there are no cures, a combination of psychological and physical therapies appear to provide significant benefits. Cognitive behavioral therapy (CBT) may provide insight into teaching relaxation techniques and stress management behaviors as well as some additional mechanisms to help cope with pain and better manage the symptoms and environment surrounding any pain syndrome. Physical, psychological, and social factors can all play a role in pain management, coping skills, attitudes, and behaviors. CBT is based on the concept or the idea that both thought and behavior patterns can affect symptoms, possibly lead to disability, and may serve as obstacles to recovery. As an example, if feelings of a familiar type of pain begin or pain symptoms become increasingly aggravated, what develops is a sense of how the pain state will continue to progress. If the previous historical recall of the pain is remembered as being severe or long lasting, then there are developed expectations that the pain will become more intense. This type of thinking can often result in feelings of being out of control or modes of helplessness that can make it seem difficult, if not impossible, to make any forward and positive progress in ever getting better. A stress response like this that often results may then trigger physical changes in the body, such as a rise in blood pressure, release of additional stress hormones, muscle tension, and more pain (whether true, escalated, or imaginary). According to the theory behind CBT, it is a type of psychotherapy based on the idea that one's own distorted

---

T.M. Halaszynski, D.M.D., M.D., M.B.A. (✉)
Department of Anesthesiology, Yale University School of Medicine and Yale-New Haven Hospital, 333 Cedar Street, P.O. Box 208051, New Haven, CT 06520-8051, USA
e-mail: Thomas.Halaszynski@yale.edu

thoughts and beliefs are what is responsible for and leads to negative moods and unhealthy behavior, all of which can impact upon pain states. CBT enforces the concept and stresses the notion that other individuals, events, or situations are not responsible for negatively altered mood and behavior. In addition, there are a host of situations in which automatic, but inaccurate, negative thoughts or beliefs are generated. These inaccurate thoughts can then often lead to unhealthy moods and behavior, such as anxiety and over-reacting (overeating behavior as an example). CBT works to interrupt the initiation or the sequence of ill feelings and negative mood shifts by making one fully aware of these inaccurate thoughts and beliefs. Therefore, CBT may then permit an individual to learn to view situations more realistically. This in turn allows the negative and runaway thoughts, behaviors, and mood to change, thus portraying an ability to behave and react in a more conscience healthy manner (even if the situation itself may not have changed). CBT is a relatively common type of psychotherapy that combines features of both cognitive therapy and behavior therapy. CBT may be helpful for numerous mental illness diseases, pain management, and other various stressful life situations.

Stress and Physical Interactions That Create Pain

Although stress can occur in so many different forms, our body tends to respond in characteristic ways that can cause, aggravate, and/or maintain pain. Physical reactions to stress can interact with chronic pain (e.g., low back, TMJ, headache, neck) in ways that are unique to that particular disorder.

Low back pain can often be aggravated by stress accompanying increases in muscle activity in the lower back. Furthermore, as with any pain, stress and mood can influence how pain information is processed and perceived. Also, with low back and arthritic pain, physical limitations often lead to bad moods, which influence the quality of life.

Temporomandibular dysfunction (TMD) patients have certain physical problems with their jaw and related muscles. During stress, which most people experience to various degrees, neck and jaw muscles become tight producing a mechanical aggravation of the painful area leading to increased pain. TMD patients often experience facial pain upon awakening which is highly correlated with grinding or clenching teeth during sleep [1].

Headache patients have physical predispositions that make them more vulnerable to normal stress levels. Physical responses to stress include increased muscle activity in the neck, disturbance of blood flow to the head, and inflammation of muscles in the neck and head. These responses often lead to headaches in the predisposed individual.

Neck pain as well as facial and head pain can be due to overactive muscles leading to inflammation known as "myofascial" pain. In response to this increased muscle activity, further inflammation occurs [2]. This creates a vicious circle where pain is maintained and increased.

Pain and stress together may result in a vicious circle where one entity can aggravate the other. The most common source of stress for a person who has pain is pain itself. Many of the above reactions can occur while feeling pain, which serves to maintain or increase pain in an upwardly spiraling cycle.

Description of Cognitive Therapy and Treatment

Overall, most CBTs have the following ten characteristics and have five typical steps involved in the conduction of such therapy (but not all may appropriately be applicable to pain disorders).

Characteristics of Cognitive Behavioral Therapy

1. CBT is based on the cognitive model of emotional response. CBT is based on the idea that our thoughts cause our feelings and behaviors, not external things, like people, situations, and events. The benefit of this fact is that we can change the way we think to feel and act better even if the situation does not change.
2. CBT is usually briefer and time limited. CBT is considered among the most rapid in terms of the results obtained. The average number of sessions patients usually receive (across all types of problems and approaches to CBT) is only 16. Other forms of therapy, like psychoanalysis, can take years. What enables CBT to be briefer is its highly instructive nature and the fact that it often makes use of homework assignments. CBT is time limited in that patients understand at the very beginning of the therapy process that there will be a point when the formal therapy will end. The ending of the formal therapy is a decision made by the therapist and patient. Therefore, CBT is not an open-ended or never-ending process for the patient and therapist.
3. A sound therapeutic relationship is necessary for effective CBT therapy, but not the focus. Some forms of therapy assume that the main reason people get better into therapy is because of the positive relationship between the therapist and patient. Cognitive behavioral therapists believe that it is important to have a good and trusting relationship, but that is not enough. CBT therapists believe that the patients change because they learn how to think differently and they act on that learning. Therefore, CBT therapists focus on teaching rational self-counseling skills for patients.
4. CBT is a collaborative effort between the therapist and patient. Cognitive behavioral therapists seek to learn what patients want out of life or the reason why patients are seeking help (their goals) and then help patients achieve those goals. The therapist's role is to listen, teach, and encourage, while the patient's role is to express concerns, learn, and implement that learning.

5. CBT is based on aspects of stoic philosophy. Not all approaches to CBT emphasize stoicism. Rational emotional behavior therapy and rational living therapy emphasize aspects of stoicism (for example: Beck's Cognitive Therapy is not based on stoicism).

    CBT does not tell people how they should feel. However, most people seeking therapy do not want to feel the way they have been feeling. The approaches that emphasize stoicism teach the benefits of feeling, at worst, calm when confronted with undesirable situations or pain conditions. They also emphasize the fact that we have our undesirable situations whether we are upset about them or not. If we are upset about our problems, we have two problems: the problem and our being upset about it. Most people want to have the fewest number of problems possible. So when we learn how to more calmly accept a personal problem, not only do we feel better, but we also usually put ourselves in a better position to make use of our intelligence, knowledge, energy, and resources to resolve the problem.

6. CBT uses the Socratic method. Cognitive behavioral therapists want to gain a very good understanding of patient concerns. That is why patients are initially asked a host of questions and why patients are encouraged to ask questions of themselves, like "How do I really know that those people are laughing at me?" and "Could they be laughing about something else?"

7. CBT is structured and directive. Cognitive behavioral therapists have a specific agenda for each session. Specific techniques and concepts are taught during each session. CBT focuses on patient goals. Patients are not told what their goals "should" be or what they "should" tolerate. CBT is directive in the sense that it shows patients how to think and behave in ways to obtain what they want. Therefore, CBT therapists do not tell patients what to do—rather, they teach patients how to do.

8. CBT is based on an educational model. CBT is based on the scientifically supported assumption that most emotional and behavioral reactions are learned. The goal of therapy is to help patients unlearn their unwanted reactions and learn a new way of reacting. Therefore, CBT has nothing to do with "just talking." The educational emphasis of CBT has an additional benefit as it can hopefully lead to long-term results for some patients. When people understand how and why they are doing well, they know what to do to continue doing well.

9. CBT theory and techniques rely on the inductive method. A central aspect of rational thinking is that it is based on fact. Often, we can upset ourselves about things when, in fact, the situation is not like we think it is. If we knew that, we would not waste our time upsetting ourselves. Therefore, the inductive method encourages us to look at our thoughts as being hypotheses or guesses that can be questioned and tested. If we find that our hypotheses are incorrect (because we have new information), then we can change our thinking to be in line with how the situation really is.

10. Homework is a central feature of CBT. If when you attempted to learn your multiplication tables you spent only 1 h per week studying them, you might still be wondering what 5×5 equals. You very likely spent a great deal of time at

Table 8.1 Cognitive behavioral therapy as a treatment modality in pain disorders

1. It is the patient's preferred treatment source or treatment modality
2. Psychiatric and antidepressant drugs are contraindicated due to adverse reactions, side effects, or allergy
3. Other treatment modalities have been tried without success
4. Other treatment options are not appropriate for a particular patient
5. Patients may wish to experience emotional growth and healing while maintaining control
6. Patients are having a hard time overcoming negative moods and self-destructive behaviors associated with their pain disorder
7. Patients want to prevent a relapse of their condition or have a mechanism to better deal with a disorder if it should return after reducing or stopping medications or other treatment modalities

home studying your multiplication tables, maybe with flash cards. The same is the case with CBT. Goal achievement (if obtained) could take a very long time if a person only practices and thinks about the techniques and topics taught was for 1 h per week. That is why CBT therapists assign reading assignments and encourage patients to practice the techniques learned on a more frequent and recurring basis.

Cognitive distortions can worsen pain states and chronic pain conditions as well as other conditions such as depression, anxiety, and phobias. Working with a trained cognitive behavioral therapist is probably the best way to learn CBT and to apply it effectively to assist in the management of pain conditions and in one's life. Used as part of a multimodal regimen, pain syndromes and pain states, depression, and anxiety can be effectively treated with CBT. Under a host of various conditions, CBT alone may not be enough depending on the severity and etiology of pain. There are several instances in which medication may be recommended along with CBT. CBT is just one type of talk therapy used to treat pain as there are numerous other effective types and treatment paradigms. Patients should confide and then consult and talk with their health care provider to find the best type or combination of treatment for a particular type of pain disorder. For CBT to be most effective, cooperation together with the patient, health care team, and counselor toward common goals is what is required.

One method of CBT for pain management is typically carried out in small group sessions of four to eight patients, and sessions are conducted weekly for 8–10 weeks. The patient-oriented group sessions are typically led by a psychologist or a psychologist–nurse educator team. CBT is one of many potential effective mechanisms to treat a wide range of life stressors, pain and pain syndromes, and mental illnesses. Table 8.1 identifies several indicators as to why CBT is performed and when to consider such behavioral therapy in pain management protocols.

Pain management modalities often result in varying degrees of success, and patient descriptions of pain can sometimes be confusing, leading to what seems to be ineffective treatment or an inability to properly identify the most appropriate course or intervention. The complexities of influences that directly and indirectly influence both pain diagnosis and pain management therapy remain unprecedented.

Table 8.2 Other conditions and issues cognitive behavioral therapy may help address

Pain disorders	Sexual disorders
Bipolar disorder	Sleep disorders
Anxiety disorders	Marital and relationship problems
Phobias	Grief and anger
Eating disorders	Depression
Substance abuse disorders	Work problems
Personality disorders	Abuse
Psychotic disorders, such as schizophrenia	Medical illnesses, such as chronic fatigue syndrome

It is also virtually impossible to separate pain-producing disorders and pain management counseling from the realities of life and living experiences. Therefore, a host of conditions and issues, in addition to pain management treatment, that CBT may help to reduce or negate their negative influences are indicated in Table 8.2. The number of issues identified in Table 8.2 must also be addressed in order to achieve maximal results from CBT for treatment of pain scenarios since they cannot be removed, but will continue to negatively influence treatment attempts. In some severe cases, CBT may be more effective when it's combined with other treatments, such as psychiatric medications.

CBT for pain management treatment modalities is based upon a cognitive behavioral model of pain [3]. A most important concept is that the hallmark of this model contains the notion that pain and pain syndromes are complex experiences that are influenced by not only underlying pathophysiology but also an individuals' cognitions, affect, and behavior [4]. CBT for pain management includes three basic components: (1) The first is a treatment rationale directed toward helping patients understand that cognitions and behavior can most certainly affect the pain experience and stresses to emphasize the role that patients can play in controlling their own pain. (2) The second component of CBT focuses on individual development and utilization of coping skills, training in psychological adaptation, and management. (3) The third component of CBT involves the application and continued maintenance of these learned coping skills.

Training can typically be provided in a wide variety of cognitive and behavioral pain coping strategies. Progressive relaxation and trigger or cue-controlled brief relaxation exercises are used to decrease muscle tension, reduce emotional distress, and divert attention away from pain or pain thoughts. Activity pacing and pleasant activity scheduling can also be used to help patients increase both the level and range of their relaxation and pleasant activity engagement. By providing patients with the appropriate tools, training in distraction techniques such as pleasant imagery, counting methods, and use of a focal point may help patients learn to divert attention away from severe pain episodes.

Another tool in the armamentarium of CBT is cognitive restructuring that is used to help patients identify and challenge overly negative pain-related thoughts and to replace these negative impressions or untoward thoughts with more adaptive, coping thoughts and skills. During the maintenance phase of learned coping skills, patients are encouraged to apply this newly learned behavior to a progressively wider range of daily situations. Patients can be provided with the skills necessary to engage in problem-solving methods that enable them to analyze and develop plans for dealing with pain flares or recurrence and other challenging situations when they begin or when pain becomes increasingly aggravating. Self-monitoring and behavioral contracting methods also are used to prompt and reinforce frequent coping skill practice. Psychological adaptation by the patient is a key factor in successful outcomes for mitigation of pain.

Although the treatment procedures of CBT described above can be used in managing acute pain, these same techniques are commonly used in the management of persistent pain [5]. In recent history, randomized, controlled studies have been carried out with a number of varying patient populations. As an example, Turner et al. demonstrated the usefulness of CBT in management of chronic low back pain, and CBT produced significant decreases in physical and psychosocial disability when compared to a waiting list control condition [6]. Several of the improvements reported by patients receiving CBT were maintained for periods of up to 12 months following treatment. Bradley et al. conducted a study of CBT in patients suffering from rheumatoid arthritis and found that CBT was superior to both a social support control and NO treatment control group in (1) reducing pain behavior, (2) decreasing intensity in disease activity, and (3) minimizing associated traits of anxiety [7]. In another early study, CBT was evaluated and identified to have great degrees of efficacy in managing osteoarthritis knee pain [8]. These authors went on to conclude that at post treatment, CBT produced significant reductions in pain and psychological disability relative to an arthritis education and standard care control conditions. Syrjala et al. have been able to demonstrate the efficacy of CBT in managing some forms of cancer-related pain [9]. Thus, a host of early evidence suggests that CBT is effective in treating both acute and chronic pain conditions such as back pain and persistent disease-related pain conditions such as arthritis and cancer.

Formal training in CBT for pain management is often available through workshops held at the American Pain Society, International Association for the Study of Pain, and the Association for the Advancement of Behavior Therapy. Several centers conducting trials of CBT also provide informal training, predoctoral training, psychology internship rotations, or postdoctoral fellowships in CBT pain management.

Five Steps (Typical) Involved in Cognitive Behavioral Therapy (Table 8.3)

Although there are different ways to conduct CBT, it typically includes five steps:

1. A patient must reflect and become aware of their thoughts, emotions, and beliefs about their situations or conditions (pain disorders). Once a patient has identified any and all associated factors and issues complicating their pain conditions, the health care provider can then encourage the patient to share their thoughts.

Table 8.3 Stages of change and a clinician's tasks

Patient's stage	Clinician's tasks
Precontemplation	Increase the patient's perception of the risks and problems associated with the current behaviors (*raise doubt*)
Contemplation	Evoke reasons for the patient to change, indicate risks of not changing; strengthen the patient's self-efficacy for change of current behavior (*tip the balance*)
Preparation	Help the patient to determine the best course of action to take in seeking change (*begin to make it happen*)
Action	Help the patient to take steps toward change (*relief*)
Maintenance	Review progress; renew motivation and commitment as needed (*sustenance*)
Relapse	Help the patient review the processes of contemplation, determination, and action without becoming stuck or demoralized because of relapse (*perseverance*)

This may include what a patient would tell themselves about an experience ("self-talk"), interpretation of the meaning of a situation, and beliefs about themselves, other people, and events. The therapist may suggest that a patient keep a journal of their thoughts and self-talk. A patient's thoughts and beliefs may be positive, negative, or neutral, or they may be rational (based on reason, logic, or facts) or irrational. As a patient continues with CBT, they then begin to explore negative or inaccurate thought patterns and work to replace these with more positive, accurate thinking.

2. A patient must try and identify troubling situations or conditions in their life. These of course include such issues as the pain disorder or other medical condition, divorce, grief, anger, and specific mental illnesses, such as panic disorder or bipolar disorder. The patient and health care provider may have to spend some time deciding what problems and goals the patient needs to focus upon.
3. Identify negative or inaccurate patient thinking: A patient's thoughts about a situation or a condition can affect the way they react to such issues. Inaccurate or negative thoughts and beliefs about something or someone can lead a patient to react in undesirable ways. To help a patient determine whether distorted thinking may be contributing to their problem, the therapist may ask the patient to pay attention to their physical, emotional, and behavioral responses to a troubling event.
4. Challenge negative or inaccurate thinking: As the patient continues to examine their thinking patterns, the therapist may encourage them to test the validity of their thoughts and beliefs. This may include asking oneself whether their view of an event fits the facts and logic and whether there might be other explanations for a situation. This step can sometimes be difficult as a patient may have long-standing ways of thinking about their life and themselves. Many thought patterns are first developed in childhood. Thoughts and beliefs that are held for a long time feel normal and correct to the patient. The patient may not easily recognize inaccuracies in their thinking.
5. A patient then needs to begin to change their thoughts and beliefs. The final step in the CBT process is to replace negative or inaccurate thinking with positive and

Table 8.4 Guidelines for managing pain

(a) Try to get your pain in perspective. Make a realistic appraisal. "In the scheme of things, how bad is my condition?"
(b) Do not fight with your symptoms as it only makes them worse. The more you accept your symptoms, the more they are likely to diminish
(c) Use various activities to refocus away from your pain. Dwelling on pain makes it more painful. Stretching, music, swimming, meditation, and other activities are important
(d) Seek a multidisciplinary approach to your problem, if necessary. Get a team of health care specialists, including a quality physician, psychotherapist, physical therapist, massage therapist, or other providers of pain management
(e) Develop a solid support system of family and friends. Also, there are many support groups in the community for people suffering from a variety of physical ailments and pain states
(f) Remember that the things we tell ourselves have an impact on our physical and emotional well-being

accurate thoughts and beliefs. By changing one's view of a situation and their view of themselves, they may be able to find more constructive ways to cope—their behavior will become less harmful or self-defeating. Changing one's thought patterns also can be difficult. Thoughts often occur spontaneously or automatically, without any effort on the part of the patient. It can be hard to control or turn off one's thoughts. Thoughts can be very powerful, and they are not always based on logic. It takes time and effort to learn how to replace distressing thoughts with rational, positive ones. A CBT therapist can help a patient recognize and challenge distorted thinking with more realistic thinking. A health care provider may also help a patient identify behaviors they wish to change and give them the chance to practice new ways to deal with situations that trigger negative, distorted thoughts.

CBT addresses the importance of realistic, healthy beliefs, attitudes, and behaviors in reducing the emotional and physical suffering associated with pain. CBT is geared toward identifying any emotional, cognitive, behavioral, physiological, and/or environmental (e.g., family, social, cultural, and societal) difficulties that might be influencing the experience of pain. Although it is rare for patients to become pain free, cognitive therapy teaches them how to reduce their pain, how to be less affected by their pain, and how to enhance functioning in various life roles (Table 8.4).

As described in some detail within this chapter, health care providers typically conduct a thorough intake interview prior to the start of therapy to obtain a clear picture of the person's presenting problems and history, including a thorough assessment of his or her pain including (1) location, (2) duration, (3) intensity, (4) frequency, (5) pain fluctuations, (6) description(s) of its, "triggers" and "alleviators" (what makes the pain worse or better), (7) patient's emotions, (8) thoughts, and behaviors when in pain, (9) personal coping efforts, (10) associated physical limitations and other consequences of pain (e.g., role limitations, financial and/or legal difficulties), (11) other psychosocial stressors that affect pain (e.g., personality, relationship issues, environment), (12) health care history including how the pain condition developed, (13) types of treatments received for pain, and (14) pain medications prescribed.

CBT sessions focus on helping patients learn to cope with their pain and their lives by learning (1) to think more realistically about their pain and other life events, (2) to relax more effectively than before (by using deep breathing techniques and relaxation exercises), (3) to manage their activities given their pain, (4) to communicate in an assertive manner with others including their physicians, family members, and friends about their pain, and (5) to solve problems related to their pain and other life stresses. The course of CBT typically starts with a focus on pain management and then moves to other concerns or issues (assuming that pain management is the primary goal of therapy). The primary target for change is a patient's negative, unrealistic thoughts, images, and beliefs about their pain; consequences of having pain; and other life stresses. Cognitive therapists also help patients identify behaviors that exacerbate pain and stress and teach patients new coping strategies as well as adaptive, healthy behaviors.

People who seek CBT for pain management are often seeking medical care for their pain as well. As a result, many people are prescribed medications to assist with pain management. Medication prescribed is often based on the diagnosis of the pain problem as well as the severity of pain experienced. For mild to moderate pain, most medical professionals prescribe non-opioid medications such as acetaminophen, nonsteroidal anti-inflammatory drugs such as ibuprofen, or cox-2 inhibitors. If the patient continues to experience pain, a non-opioid–opioid combination of medication is considered next. The strength of a narcotic medication (i.e., opioids) is not as important as it was once thought, because addiction comprised psychological dependence as well as a physiological process. Therefore, many physicians prescribe opioids (i.e., schedule-2) to get pain patients comfortable immediately. Adjuvant medications may also be prescribed as well. An adjuvant medication is one that has FDA approval for one area of treatment, may also have off-label uses in pain. For example, some antidepressants approved for the treatment of depression are also effective in treating neuropathic pain (based on pain research findings). The FDA has not approved it for this purpose, but they are often prescribed for such purposes because there is empirical and clinical evidence to support its use. If the patient is suffering from moderate to severe pain, many medical professionals prescribe opioids right away as well as adjuvant medications.

CBT is an effective form of treatment for people who have pain, and there is firm evidence in the research literature that CBTs are effective in reducing patient's pain levels, use of pain medications, negative thoughts, and extent of physical disability as well as enhancing a patient's pain control, emotions, physical functioning, health status, and relationships with others compared to not being in therapy at all [10, 11]. In addition, multidisciplinary pain treatment programs that incorporated CBT and behavioral therapy approaches were significantly more successful than programs that used only one treatment or programs with no other alternative treatments [12, 13]. Overall, it appears that the CBT approach has a positive effect when combined with active treatments such as medications, physical therapy, and medical treatments for chronic pain clients in treating pain, thoughts about pain, and pain behavior problems.

CBT: Why Is It Performed and What Are the Risks

The goal of CBT is to change the way a patient thinks about pain so that both their body and mind respond better during episodes of pain. Avoid dwelling on the pain state and other negative aspects. Overall the concept is simple and helps the patient to understand how their thinking can affect their mood and how thoughts in their head can affect the way they feel, which can then affect behaviors. Whatever the goals and reasons for seeking help from debilitating pain syndromes and pain states, it is clear that CBT can be helpful for some people who have acute and chronic persistent pain. CBT has virtually none of the side effects that other treatments, such as medications, can cause, and in fact, there is very little to no risk associated with CBT.

Cognitive behavioral skills can change the way a patient's mind influences their body. When a patient is able to shift their thinking away from the pain and change their focus to more positive aspects within their life, they change the way their body responds to the anticipated pain and stress. CBT can be helpful for chronic pain by changing the way a patient thinks about pain. It also teaches a patient how to become more active [14]. This helps, because pain can also improve with appropriate physical activity, such as walking or swimming.

A patient can experience pain condition(s) and may start focusing on their associated depression as well as have a thought(s) such as "I got up late this morning, so now my whole day is ruined." This thought can be the spark that gets the fire burning. The same thing can often happen in your head when you are alone. Fuel is added by thinking, "I have pain," "I am depressed," and "I can't even get up on time, what use am I to myself or others?" The negative thoughts feed on themselves. Patients will continue talking negatively to themselves, and ultimately they focus on the pain condition, allow themselves to feel more depressed, and exaggerate the circumstances and environment that they have created.

There above thought processes are also often very inaccurate. Inaccurate thoughts are also called "cognitive distortions." These negative and inaccurate thoughts can be so ingrained that they become "core beliefs" that an individual may begin to live by. An example is "I've never been successful at anything, so why even try?" Thus, CBT therapy focuses on changing a patient's thoughts about pain and illness and then helps them adopt positive ways of coping with these conditions [15].

In general, CBT poses little risk(s); however, because therapy can explore painful feelings and experiences, a patient may feel emotionally uncomfortable at times during group or individual (one-to-one) therapy. The coping skills a patient can learn should help them to later on manage and conquer distressful feelings and thoughts. Some forms of CBT, such as exposure therapy, may require a patient to confront situations that they would otherwise rather avoid (such as airplanes if you have a fear of flying). These particular situations can lead to temporary distress or anxiety, but it is not usually a direct effect of CBT in the situation of therapy for pain states and pain conditions.

CBT may not cure a patient's pain condition or make an otherwise unpleasant situation go away. However, CBT overall is a highly effective treatment, and many patients can benefit from such efforts synthesized with other pain management modalities. CBT can give a patient the power to better cope with their situation in a healthy way and to feel better about themselves and their life [16]. Many of the benefits of CBT can help a patient: (1) gain a better understanding of their pain condition or situation(s) adversely affecting their pain state, (2) help a patient to identify and change behaviors or thoughts that negatively affect their pain condition and their life, (3) explore relationships and experiences that may be adversely affecting a patient's pain disorder, (4) provide patients with an ability to find better ways to cope with pain conditions and to solve problems, (5) permit patients to learn how to set realistic goals for their life related to their pain disorder, (6) permit patients to begin to feel better about themselves, and (7) reduce the likelihood of a relapse or an exaggeration of painful conditions and pain disorders.

Acknowledgement None declared.

Conflict of Interest None declared.

References

1. Uppgaard R. Taking control of TMJ: your total wellness program for recovering from temporomandibular joint pain, whiplash, fibromyalgia, and related disorders. Oakland, CA: New Harbinger; 1999.
2. Starlanyl D, Copeland M. Fibromyalgia and chronic myofascial pain syndrome: a survival manual. Oakland, CA: New Harbinger; 1996.
3. Turk D, Meichenbaum D, Genest M. Pain and behavioral medicine: a cognitive-behavioral perspective. New York: Guilford Press; 1983.
4. Keefe FJ, Beaupre PM, Gil KM. Behavioral concepts in the analysis of chronic pain syndromes. J Consult Clin Psychol. 1986;54:776–83.
5. Jay SM, Elliot CH, Ozolins M, et al. Behavioral management of children's distress during painful medical procedures. Behav Res Ther. 1985;23:513–20.
6. Turner JA, Clancy S. Comparison of operant-behavioral and cognitive-behavioral group treatment for chronic low back pain. J Consult Clin Psychol. 1988;58:573–9.
7. Bradley LA, Young LD, Anderson JO, et al. Effects of psychological therapy on pain behavior of rheumatoid arthritis patients: treatment outcome and six-month follow-up. Arthritis Rheum. 1987;30:1105–14.
8. Keefe FJ, Caldwell DS, Williams DA, et al. Pain coping skills training in the management of osteoarthritic knee pain: a comparative study. Behav Ther. 1990;21:49–62.
9. Syrjala KL, Donaldson GW, Davies MW, et al. Relaxation and imagery and cognitive-behavioral training reduce pain during cancer treatment: a controlled clinical trial. Pain. 1995; 63:189–98.
10. Morley S, Eccleston C, Williams A. Systematic review and meta-analysis of randomized controlled trials of cognitive behaviour therapy and behaviour therapy for chronic pain in adults, excluding headache. Pain. 1999;80(1–2):1–13.
11. Van Tulder M, Ostelo R, Vlaeyen J, et al. Behavioral treatment for chronic low back pain. Spine. 2000;26:270–81.
12. Cutler R, Fishbain D, Rosomoff H, et al. Does nonsurgical pain center treatment of chronic pain return patients to work? A review and meta-analysis of the literature. Spine. 1994;19: 643–52.

13. Flor H, Fydrich T, Turk D. Efficacy of multidisciplinary pain treatment centers: a meta-analytic review. Pain. 1992;49:221–30.
14. Max MB. Pain. In: Goldman L, Ausiello D, editors. Cecil medicine. 23rd ed. Philadelphia, PA: WB Saunders Co.; 2008. p. 151–9.
15. Judith A, Turner S, et al. Mediators, moderators, and predictors of therapeutic change in cognitive-behavioral therapy for chronic pain. Pain. 2007;127:276–86.
16. Gatchel RJ, Turk DC. Psychological approaches to pain management: a practitioner's handbook. New York: Guilford; 2010.

Chapter 9
Management of Oral Ulcers and Burning Mouth Syndrome

Thomas M. Halaszynski

Definitions

Oral Ulcers

Mouth ulcers (aphthae) and the syndrome of burning mouth are common and due to a host of both systemic and iatrogenic causes (Tables 9.1 and 9.2). Mouth ulcers are most commonly due to trauma such as from fractured teeth, ill-fitting dentures and partials, or dental (tooth) fillings. Patients with aphthae are usually otherwise healthy, but systemic diseases that should be excluded include Behcet's syndrome, gluten-sensitive enteropathy, deficiencies of hematinics, celiac disease [1], and, occasionally, immunodeficiency. However, patients with an oral ulcer present with duration of 3 weeks or greater should be referred for biopsy of the oral lesion or other investigations to exclude possible malignancy or additional serious conditions such as chronic infections. Both treatment and management strategies may vary depending upon the determined etiology of the aphthous ulcers. Therapies are often directed toward resolution of symptoms unless a definitive systemic cause of ulcer development can be identified. Recurrent aphthous stomatitis is a clinical diagnosis, and predisposing factors should be identified and corrected [2]. Subsequent to removal of the cause or irritating etiology, oral ulcers related to trauma usually resolve in about a week.

Ulcerative conditions, such as aphthous stomatitis, can typically begin in childhood or adolescence with recurrent small, round, or ovoid oral ulcers, usually with well-circumscribed margins, yellow or grey floors, and erythematous haloes (Fig. 9.1). Oral ulcers develop on soft tissues in the mouth and at the base of the gums. These oral lesions occur singly or in clusters on the inside surfaces of the cheeks or

---

T.M. Halaszynski, D.M.D., M.D., M.B.A. (✉)
Department of Anesthesiology, Yale University School of Medicine and Yale-New Haven Hospital, 333 Cedar Street, P.O. Box 208051, New Haven, CT 06520-8051, USA
e-mail: Thomas.Halaszynski@yale.edu

Table 9.1 Main systemic and iatrogenic causes of oral ulcers

Microbial disease	Malignant neoplasms
Herpetic stomatitis	Blood disorders
Chicken pox	Anemia
Herpes zoster	Leukemia
Hand, foot, and mouth disease	Neutropenia
Herpangina	Other white cell dyscrasias
Infectious mononucleosis	Gastrointestinal disease
HIV infection	Celiac disease
Acute necrotizing gingivitis	Crohn's disease
Tuberculosis	Ulcerative colitis
Syphilis	Rheumatoid disease
Fungal infections	Lupus erythematosus
Cutaneous disease	Behcet's disease
Lichen planus	Sweet's syndrome
Pemphigus	Reiter's disease
Pemphigoid	Drugs
Erythema multiforme	Cytotoxic agents
Dermatitis herpetiformis	Nicorandil
Linear IgA disease	Others
Epidermolysis bullosa	
Chronic ulcerative stomatitis	
Other dermatoses	
Radiotherapy	

Patients with a mouth ulcer lasting over 3 weeks should be referred for biopsy or other investigations to exclude malignancy or other serious conditions

Table 9.2 Main causes of burning mouth syndrome

Dry mouth (xerostomia)	Caused by medications or other health problems
Dentures	Dentures can place stress on muscles and tissues of the mouth causing mouth pain. Materials used in dentures can irritate tissues in the mouth
Nutritional deficiencies	Lack of zinc, folate, iron, thiamine, riboflavin, cobalamin, pyridoxine
Allergy or reactions	To foods, food flavorings, food additives, fragrances, dyes, or others
Psychological factors	Anxiety, health worries, depression
Reflux disease	Stomach acid (gastroesophageal reflux disease) that enters the mouth from the upper gastrointestinal tract
Medication(s)	Particularly high blood pressure medications called angiotensin-converting enzyme (ACE) inhibitors
Endocrine disorders	Such as diabetes and underactive thyroid (hypothyroidism)
Hormonal imbalance	Such as those associated with menopause
Excessive mouth irritation	May result from overbrushing of tongue, overuse of mouthwashes, or too many acidic drinks
Oral habits	Such as tongue thrusting and teeth grinding (bruxism)
Nerve damage	To nerves that control taste and pain in the tongue
Others or unknown	Oral yeast infection (thrush), oral lichen planus, and geographic tongue

Fig. 9.1 Oral ulcer of the lower lip

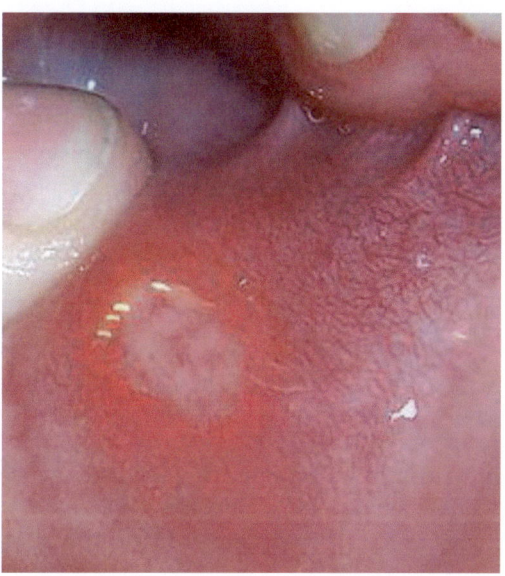

lips, on or under tongue, at the base of the gingiva, or on the soft palate [3]. Unlike cold sores/blisters, mouth ulcers do not occur on the surface of the lips and are not contagious. These oral ulcerative conditions can be very painful and can make eating and talking difficult.

Most oral ulcers will heal and disappear within a week or two. Unusually large or painful mouth ulcers or ulcers that do not seem to heal should be further investigated and/or biopsied. Aphthous stomatitis affects at least 20 % of the population, and its natural course is one of eventual remission. There are three main clinical types: (1) minor aphthous ulcers (80 % of all aphthae), (2) major aphthous ulcers, and (3) herpetiform ulcers.

Trench mouth, formally known as Vincent's stomatitis, acute necrotizing ulcerative gingivitis, and necrotizing ulcerative gingivitis, is a severe form of gingivitis that causes painful, infected, bleeding gums, but may also be a cause of oral ulcerations. Although trench mouth is rare in developed nations, it remains common in several developing countries with poor nutrition and poor living conditions. Trench mouth earned its common nickname because of its prevalence among soldiers who were stuck in the trenches during World War I without the means to take care of their teeth properly.

Burning Mouth Syndrome

Burning mouth syndrome (BMS) is a common yet complex problem that causes chronic burning pain in the mouth and/or tongue. Pain from BMS can affect the tongue, gums, lips, inside the cheeks, roof of the mouth, or widespread areas of the whole mouth [4]. There are often no visible signs of irritation. Pain can sometimes be severe, as if the mouth was scalded. Often the cause of BMS cannot be determined which makes treatment more difficult, but BMS can usually be kept under control [5]. The cause of the syndrome may be due to the onset of menopause or to vitamin deficiencies. About 5 % of the population, usually people over the age of 60, are affected with this condition. It often occurs more frequently in older women, often in menopausal women. Some other names for BMS include scalded mouth syndrome, burning tongue syndrome, burning lips syndrome, glossodynia, and stomatodynia.

BMS can often have features of a neuropathy [6] and could be related to the production of toxic free radicals that are released in stress situations. Alpha-lipoic acid is an antioxidant able to increase the levels of intracellular glutathione and eliminate free radicals. Femiano et al. found that following treatment with alpha-lipoic acid, there was a significant symptomatic improvement compared with placebo, with the majority showing at least some improvement after 2 months, thus supporting the hypothesis that BMS is a neuropathy [7].

Symptoms

Oral Ulcers

Patients may notice a tingling or burning sensation a day or two before aphthous ulcer(s) actually appear. There are several types of oral ulcers, including minor, major, and herpetiform sores. Minor aphthous ulcer sores are the most common [8]: (1) are less than about 1/2 in. or 12 mm in diameter, (2) are oval shaped, and (3) typically heal without scarring in 1–2 weeks. Major aphthous ulcer lesions are less common: (1) are greater than about 1/2 in. or 12 mm in diameter, (2) have irregular edges, (3) typically heal slowly and may take up to 6 weeks, and (4) can often leave extensive scarring. Herpetiform aphthous ulcer sores usually develop later in life: (1) are each no bigger than about 1/8 in. or 3 mm in diameter, (2) often occur in multiple pinpoint ulcer clusters of 10–100 sores, (3) have irregular edges, and (4) heal without scarring in 1–4 weeks.

Additional symptoms patients may experience along with the oral lesions include fever, listlessness, and swollen lymph nodes. Patients should be instructed to consult a doctor if they experience any of the following symptoms: (1) unusually large aphthous ulcers; (2) recurring ulcers, with new ones developing before old ones heal; (3) persistent sores lasting 3 weeks or more; (4) sores that extend into the lips themselves (vermilion border); (5) pain that cannot be controlled by self-care measures, (6) extreme difficulty eating and/or drinking, and (7) evidence of high fever in conjunction with aphthous ulcer lesions.

Burning Mouth Syndrome

Symptoms of BMS and mouth ulcers may include [9] (1) a burning sensation that may affect your tongue, lips, gums, palate, throat, or whole mouth; (2) a tingling or a numb sensation in your mouth or on the tip of your tongue; (3) mouth pain that may worsen as the day progresses; (4) a sensation of dry mouth and increased thirst; (5) sore mouth and loss of taste; and (6) taste changes, such as a bitter or metallic taste.

The pain from BMS may show several patterns. It may occur every day, with little pain in the morning and becoming worse as the day progresses. It may start upon awakening and last all day. Or the pain may come and go, and there may even be some entirely pain-free days. Whatever the pattern of mouth pain that may occur, BMS symptoms often last for years before proper diagnosis and treatment are rendered. In some cases, symptoms may suddenly go away on their own or become less frequent. BMS usually does not cause any noticeable physical changes to the tongue (except for geographic tongue) or the mouth (except for lichen planus, thrush, or oral yeast infection) [10].

Risk Factors

Oral Ulcers

Anyone can develop oral ulcers, but certain factors can make one more susceptible. Females are more susceptible to aphthous stomatitis, especially the development of clusters of small lesions as they are more common in women [11]. About one-third of patients with recurrent oral ulcer development have a strong family history of the disorder. This observation may be due to heredity or a shared factor(s) in the environment, such as certain foods or allergens.

Burning Mouth Syndrome

Typically, BMS is uncommon but generally starts later in life in the 50s, 60s, or 70s. It usually affects women more frequently and may begin spontaneously, with no known triggering factor(s). Some research studies suggest that certain factors may increase the risk of developing BMS, and these risk factors may include: (1) the so-called supertaster, an individual with a high density of small tongue papillae which contain taste buds [12]; (2) upper respiratory tract infection; (3) previous dental procedures; (4) allergic reactions to food or medications [13]; and (5) traumatic life events or stress.

Complications

Oral Ulcers

Oral ulcers often recur, but they may be able to be reduced in frequency by addressing factors that seem to trigger their occurrence [14]. Certain foods can irritate the mouth (nuts, chips, pretzels, certain spices, salty foods, and acidic fruits such as pineapple, grapefruit, and oranges), stimulate ulcer development, and aggravate preexisting oral lesions. To help prevent nutritional deficiencies as a potential inciting cause of ulcer occurrence, eat plenty of fruits, vegetables, and whole grains [15]. Regularly eating yogurt that contains acidophilus or other beneficial bacteria also may help reduce or prevent aphthous ulcer development.

Complications that can trigger aphthous ulcers or further irritate oral lesions are by chewing and talking at the same time. This may cause minor trauma to the delicate lining of the mouth. Poor oral hygiene habits may aggravate or incite the development of oral ulcers. Therefore, regular brushing after meals and flossing once a day can keep the mouth clean and free of foods that might trigger oral ulcer development. Use a soft brush to help prevent irritation to delicate mouth tissues, and avoid toothpastes and mouth rinses that contain sodium lauryl sulfate [16–19]. Braces or other dental appliances can elicit or irritate oral ulcers, but the latter can be reduced or eliminated with orthodontic waxes to cover any sharp edges.

Burning Mouth Syndrome

Most of the complications that BMS may cause or associated with are mainly related to pain and include issues such as: (1) difficulty sleeping, (2) irritability, (3) depression, (4) anxiety, (5) difficulty eating or weight loss, and (6) decreased socializing activities.

Tests and Diagnosis

Oral Ulcers

Tests are not typically required or needed to diagnose aphthous ulcers. Oral lesions of aphthous ulcer origin can be identified simply with a visual examination. Under certain circumstances, specified tests are performed to check for other health problems, especially if the aphthous ulcers are severe and ongoing [20].

A complete medical history and oral facial examination must be performed to first determine the differential diagnosis of oral facial pain from oral ulcers and from symptoms of pain in the mouth from ulcers. The history should inquire about

Table 9.3 History of soft tissue oral facial pain

Chief complaint(s)			
Pain location			
Pain onset	Progression	Association with other factors	
Pain characteristics (and concomitant symptoms)	Pain quality(s)	Intensity and flow of pain	Pain behavior: duration, frequency, temporal
Aggravating and alleviating factors	Medications and physical modalities	Function and parafunction	Sleep disturbances and emotional stress
Past consultation and/or treatment	Relationship to other patient complaints		

Table 9.4 Examination of soft tissue oral facial pain

General examination	Vital signs	Blood pressure and pulse	Respiratory rate and temperature
	Cranial nerve examination	Balance and coordination	
	Eye, ear, and cervical evaluation		
Muscle exam	Palpation	Pain and tenderness	Trigger points and pain referral
Mastication evaluation	Range of mandibular movement	Measurement	Pain
	TMJ evaluation	Pain	Dysfunction
	Oral structures	Teeth and occlusion	Mucogingival tissues Periodontium
Other diagnostic tests	Imaging	Laboratory tests	Psychologic provocation tests

TMJ temporomandibular joint

details related to the chief complaint(s) and characteristics of the pain (Table 9.3). In addition to a past medical history, complete review of symptoms and a psychosocial assessment should be performed. The clinical oral examination should be directed toward identifying the origin of the intraoral pain and direct examination of any oral ulcers (Table 9.4). Use of benzydamine hydrochloride 0.15 % mouthwash or spray may provide symptomatic relief, and continued use of chlorhexidine 0.2 % aqueous mouthwash can help maintain good oral hygiene along with proper and continued tooth brushing [21]. Topical corticosteroids aid resolution of ulcers, and in severe cases systemic immunomodulation may be needed.

Burning Mouth Syndrome

There is no single test that can determine if BMS is present or what may be causing mouth pain. Usually the first course of action is to try and rule out other probable

Table 9.5 Diagnostic tests for burning mouth syndrome(s)

Blood tests	Blood tests to check complete blood count, glucose level, thyroid function, nutritional factors, and immune functioning
Oral cultures	Cultures from the mouth to diagnose fungal, bacterial, or viral infection
Imaging	MRI, CT scan, or other imaging checking for other health problems
Allergy tests	Allergy testing to determine allergy to certain foods, additives, or substances in denture construction
Salivary measurements	Salivary tests can confirm whether there is reduced salivary flow
Gastric reflux tests	To determine the presence of gastroesophageal reflux disease (GERD)
Psychological questionnaire	To determine symptoms of depression, anxiety, or other mental health conditions

problems before diagnosing BMS. This can be accomplished by performing a medical history, identifying all medications (and medications recently taken or stopped), examining the mouth, determining the description of symptoms, and identifying any abnormal oral habits and oral care routines. In addition, performance of a general medical examination is warranted for signs of other medical conditions (Tables 9.3 and 9.4).

A consideration or part of the diagnostic process may include some of the following tests identified in Table 9.5. In addition, if there is strong suspicion that medication(s) may contribute to mouth pain, it may be suggested to temporarily stop the potential offending medication(s) if possible to determine if the pain lessens or becomes eliminated. Caution should always be exercised before holding medication(s) and proper medical advice obtained since it can be dangerous to stop some medicines [13].

Treatments and Drugs

Oral Ulcers

Treatment is usually not necessary for minor aphthous ulcers that tend to clear spontaneously within a week or two. Large, persistent, or unusually painful aphthous ulcer lesions often require medical care [20, 22]. A number of treatment options exist, ranging from mouth rinses and topical ointments to systemic corticosteroids for the most severe cases [23] (Table 9.6).

There are several relatively simple treatment options to alleviate symptoms from oral ulcers, relieve pain, and speed healing. These modalities could include: (1) mouth rinsing using salt water; baking soda (dissolve 1 teaspoon of baking soda in 1/2 cup warm water); hydrogen peroxide diluted by half with water; a mixture of 1 part diphenhydramine (Benadryl) to either 1 part bismuth subsalicylate (Kaopectate) or 1 part simethicone (Maalox), and (2) protection of the oral lesions until healed by covering them with a paste made of baking soda or use of over-the-counter products that contain a numbing agent (Anbesol and Orajel).

Table 9.6 Treatment options for oral ulcers

Mouth rinses	A mouth rinse containing the steroid dexamethasone may reduce pain and inflammation (prescribed in conditions of multiple numbers of oral lesions). Oral suspensions of the antibiotic tetracycline may also reduce pain and healing time (tetracycline has potential drawbacks: make patients more susceptible to oral thrush (fungal infection) and may permanently discolor children's teeth)
Topical pastes	Over-the-counter and prescription pastes with active ingredients such as benzocaine (Orabase), amlexanox (Aphthasol), and fluocinonide (Lidex, Vanos) can relieve pain and speed healing if applied to individual lesions as soon as they appear
Oral medications	Medications such as the heartburn drug cimetidine (Tagamet) and colchicine (Tx of gout) may be helpful for mouth ulcer sores. Oral steroid medications can be prescribed when severe oral ulcers do not respond to other treatments (since the side effects of steroids can be serious, they are usually considered a treatment of last resort)
Debacterol	This topical solution is designed to treat oral ulcers and gingival lesions by chemically cauterizing them, and it reduces healing time to about a week
Nutritional supplements	Nutritional supplements are needed when there are low amounts of important nutrients, such as folate (folic acid), vitamin B-6, vitamin B-12, and zinc
Others	When oral ulcers are related to other more serious health problems, the underlying condition requires treatment

Additional measures to consider as simple treatment options to alleviate symptoms from oral ulcers include: (1) avoiding abrasive, acidic, or spicy foods that can cause further irritation and pain; (2) apply ice to the oral ulcer(s) or allow ice chips to slowly dissolve over the lesions; (3) brush teeth gently, using a soft brush and toothpaste without foaming agents (e.g., TheraBreath); and (4) dab a small amount of milk of magnesia on the oral ulcer a few times daily (this may ease the pain and help the sore heal more quickly).

There are several drug-free options to consider for treating and preventing aphthous ulcers, including nutritional supplements (including zinc [24], folate, and vitamin B [25]), a paste of alum, slippery elm powder, or deglycyrrhizinated licorice (DGL) applied directly to the lesion and stress reduction techniques, such as yoga and meditation.

Burning Mouth Syndrome

Currently, there is no single definitive treatment or modality to treat BMS, and research on the most effective method(s) has not been determined [26, 27]. Treatment depends on the particular signs and symptoms as well as identifying any underlying conditions that may be causing burning mouth pain. It remains important to try and diagnose what may be causing burning mouth pain, and once any underlying causes are treated, BMS symptoms typically improve [12, 28]. There is no known way to prevent BMS, but by taking measures to avoid acidic foods and drinks < tobacco <

Table 9.7 Treatment options for burning mouth syndrome

Clonazepam (Klonopin)	A lozenge-type form of an anticonvulsant medication
Alpha-lipoic acid	An antioxidant produced naturally by the body
Oral thrush medications	If cultures determine an infectious etiology
Certain antidepressants	When diagnosis of depression has been identified
B vitamins	If diagnosis of vitamin deficiency has been determined
Cognitive behavioral therapy	Psychological or psychiatric consultation may be necessary
Special oral rinses or mouth washes	Typically to treat symptoms or to remove any potential aggravating etiologies
Saliva replacement products	Used when the cause is diagnosed from reduced salivary production
Capsaicin	A pain reliever that comes from chili peppers
Surgery	Surgery is not typically recommended for burning mouth syndrome

and reduce stress, a patient may be able to reduce the pain from BMS or prevent mouth pain from becoming worse [29].

If an etiology for a diagnosis of BMS is not determined (truly idiopathic), treatment can prove to be challenging. There is currently no known cure for primary BMS, and several treatment methods or modalities may need to be implemented before finding one or a combination of therapies that may be helpful in reducing burning mouth pain. Treatment options for BMS are identified in Table 9.7.

In addition to the medical treatment and any prescription medications indicated (Table 9.7), additional measures may help to improve symptoms from BMS. Several self-help measures may also prove beneficial for reducing chronic mouth pain and include: (1) drinking more fluids to ease the feeling of dry mouth; (2) avoiding the use of any tobacco products; (3) avoiding products containing cinnamon or mint; (4) avoiding spicy hot foods; (5) avoiding acidic foods and liquids, such as tomatoes, orange juice, soft drinks, and coffee; (6) changing to a different brand of toothpaste; and (7) exercising measures to reduce excessive life stresses.

It must be remembered that BMS can be painful and very frustrating for patients, especially since it may take months or years for a patient to seek and receive a diagnosis and effective treatment. In addition, BMS can reduce the quality of life if a patient does not take steps to remain positive and stay hopeful. There are some measures or suggested techniques to help patients cope with BMS such as: (1) practicing relaxation exercises (yoga), (2) joining a pain support group, (3) engaging in pleasurable activities (such as exercise or hobbies), and (4) making efforts to stay socially active and connecting with family and friends.

Acknowledgement None declared.

Conflict of Interest None declared.

References

1. Sedghizadeh P, Shuler C, Allen C, et al. Celiac disease and recurrent aphthous stomatitis: a report and review of the literature. Oral Surg Oral Med Oral Pathol Oral Radiol Endod. 2002;94(4):474–8.
2. Jurge S, Kuffer R, Scully C, et al. Mucosal disease series. Number VI. Recurrent aphthous stomatitis. Oral Dis. 2006;12(1):1–21.
3. Bruce A, Rogers R. Acute oral ulcers. Dermatol Clin. 2003;21(1):1–15.
4. James W, Berger T et al. In: Andrews' diseases of the skin: clinical dermatology. Saunders Elsevier; 2006; 57. ISBN 0-7216-2921-0.
5. Grushka M, Kawalec J, Epstein J. Burning mouth syndrome: evolving concepts. Oral Maxillofac Surg Clin North Am. 2000;12:287–95.
6. Bartoshuk L, Grushka M, Duffy V, et al. Burning mouth syndrome: damage to CN VII and pain phantoms in CN V. Chem Senses. 1999;24:609.
7. Femiano F, Gombos F, Scully C. Burning mouth syndrome: open trial of psychotherapy alone, medication with alpha-lipoic acid (thioctic acid), and combination therapy. Med Oral. 2004; 9(1):8–13.
8. Scully, Crispian (2008). Oral and maxillofacial medicine : the basis of diagnosis and treatment (2nd ed. ed.). Edinburgh: Churchill Livingstone. pp. 171–175. ISBN 9780443068188.
9. Grushka M, Epstein JB, Gorsky M. Burning mouth syndrome. Am Fam Physician. 2002;65(4):615–20.
10. De Rossi S, Greenberg M. Intraoral contact allergy: a literature review and case reports. J Am Dent Assoc. 1998;129(10):1435–41.
11. McCartan B, Sullivan A. The association of menstrual cycle, pregnancy, and menopause with recurrent oral aphthous stomatitis: a review and critique. Obstet Gynecol. 1992;80(3):455–8.
12. Femiano F, Gombos F, Esposito V, et al. Burning mouth syndrome (BMS): evaluation of thyroid and taste. Med Oral Patol Oral Cir Bucal. 2006;11(1):E22–5.
13. Brown R, Krakow A, Douglas T, et al. 'Scalded mouth syndrome' caused by angiotensin converting enzyme inhibitors. Oral Surg Oral Med Oral Pathol Oral Radiol Endod. 1997;83:665–7.
14. Ussher M, West R, Stepto A, et al. Increase in common cold symptoms and mouth ulcers following smoking cessation. Tob Control. 2003;12(1):86–8.
15. Wray D, Ferguson M, Hutcheon W, et al. Nutritional deficiencies in recurrent aphthae. J Oral Pathol. 1978;7(6):418–23.
16. Herlofson B, Barkvoll P. Sodium lauryl sulfate and recurrent aphthous ulcers. A preliminary study. Acta Odontol Scand. 1994;52(5):257–9.
17. Herlofson B, Barkvoll P. The effect of two toothpaste detergents on the frequency of recurrent aphthous ulcers. Acta Odontol Scand. 1996;54(3):150–3.
18. Chahine L, Sempson N, Wagoner C. The effect of sodium lauryl sulfate on recurrent aphthous ulcers: a clinical study. Compend Contin Educ Dent. 1997;18(12):1238–40.
19. Healy C, Paterson M, Joyston-Bechal S, et al. The effect of a sodium lauryl sulfate-free dentifrice on patients with recurrent oral ulceration. Oral Dis. 1999;5(1):39–43.
20. Scully C, Shotts R. ABC of oral health. Mouth ulcers and other causes of orofacial soreness and pain. BMJ. 2000;321(7254):162–5.
21. Meiller T, Kutcher M, Overholser C, et al. Effect of an antimicrobial mouthrinse on recurrent aphthous ulcerations. Oral Surg Oral Med Oral Pathol. 1991;72(4):425–9.
22. Scully C. Clinical practice. Aphthous ulceration. N Engl J Med. 2006;355(2):165–72.
23. Barrons R. Treatment strategies for recurrent oral aphthous ulcers. Am J Health Syst Pharm. 2001;58(1):41–50. quiz 51–3.
24. Orbak R, Cicek Y, Tezel A, et al. Effects of zinc treatment in patients with recurrent aphthous stomatitis. Dent Mater J. 2003;22(1):21–9.

25. Volkov I, Rudoy I, Freud T, et al. Effectiveness of vitamin B12 in treating recurrent aphthous stomatitis: a randomized, double-blind, placebo-controlled trial. J Am Board Fam Med. 2009;22(1):9–16.
26. Woda A, Navez M, Picard P, et al. A possible therapeutic solution for stomatodynia (burning mouth syndrome). J Orofac Pain. 1998;12:272–8.
27. Maltsman-Tseikhin A, Moricca P, Niv D. Burning mouth syndrome: will better understanding yield better management? Pain Pract. 2007;7(2):151–62.
28. Femiano F, Lanza A, Buonaiuto C, et al. Burning mouth syndrome and burning mouth in hypothyroidism: proposal for a diagnostic and therapeutic protocol. Oral Surg Oral Med Oral Pathol Oral Radiol Endod. 2008;105(1):e22–7.
29. Suarez P, Clark T. Burning mouth syndrome: an update on diagnosis and treatment methods. J Calif Dent Assoc. 2006;34(8):611–22.

Chapter 10
Hypnosis and Biofeedback for Orofacial Pain Management

Janet Crain

Introduction

Today, more medical professionals are becoming interested in the mind/body connection, particularly as it relates to healing. Concerns with side effects and immunities to the effectiveness of pain medications make it difficult to treat patients with pharmaceuticals, hypnosis and biofeedback are making a resurgence in medical protocol.

In 1986, Dr. Earl Bakken defined cyberphysiology as the study of how neurally mediated autonomic responses can be modified by a learning process. Both hypnosis and biofeedback are cyberphysiologic strategies that enable the patient to develop voluntary control of certain physiologic processes [1]. Several studies have examined the effectiveness of hypnosis and biofeedback in both acute and chronic pain management.

My Introduction to Hypnosis

My own first experience with hypnosis was both dramatic and very personal, and it quickly showed me how effective hypnosis can be for managing pain and discomfort. In 2003, I was diagnosed with a recurrence of non-Hodgkin's lymphoma, cancer of the lymphatic system. I had already endured a round of radiation treatments during my first bout with lymphoma. The chemotherapy treatments to treat the recurrence caused me to lose my hair as well as 16 lb as a result of extreme nausea. My mouth became as dry as a desert, and I could hardly swallow. So, before I faced another round of chemotherapy, my husband suggested I try hypnosis to control the side effects.

J. Crain, D.M.D. (✉)
The Center for Headaches, Facial Pain, and Sleep Apnea,
2045 Route 35 South, South Amboy, NJ 08879, USA
e-mail: Drcdrk@aol.com

Most of the time, my nausea started a few hours after each chemotherapy treatment. Using hypnosis, I was able to focus my attention on replacing the nausea with hunger. After my first 45-min hypnosis session, I was amazed that it worked—the nausea disappeared, and I felt hungry instead. I also used hypnotic focus to imagine a lemon in my mouth, which increased my saliva flow, preventing the severe dry mouth I had previously experienced.

During the next 6 months of treatment, I had two to three hypnosis sessions per week to strengthen the positive empowering thoughts that helped me to counteract the side effects. The nurses and physicians who administered the chemotherapy treatment remarked repeatedly that they had never seen anyone require so little anti-nausea medication during this particular chemotherapy regimen.

Obviously, hypnosis changed my life on a deeply personal level, and since then, it has significantly changed my dental practice, which is devoted to the treatment of headaches, facial pain, and temporomandibular joint (TMJ) disorder. I was so impressed with the control that hypnosis offered me that I trained to become a certified hypnotist, which allows me to use hypnotic focus with my patients. I have modified the techniques I learned to make them chairside friendly and have incorporated them into my treatment protocol, helping my patients not only manage pain but also overcome fears and achieve relaxation.

What Hypnosis Is

In 1855, Scottish physician and surgeon James Braid coined the term "hypnotism" and essentially founded hypnotherapy as we know it today. Hypnosis can be defined as a state of heightened concentration or focused attention that allows you to tap into the extraordinary power of the mind. Contrary to popular belief, there is nothing strange or magical about hypnosis; it occurs naturally. Television and movies have misrepresented hypnosis and given it a poor reputation that is absolutely unfounded.

In fact, most of us are in a hypnotic state at various times on a daily basis. For example, you have no doubt driven home on autopilot, so deep in thought that you had no recollection of the drive before arriving in your parking spot. While reading, you may sometimes lose track of time and fail to notice someone walking into the room because you are so engrossed in your book. These are all examples of a hypnotic trance state. In this state, you become more relaxed, focused, and suggestible. What we usually call "daydreaming" is also a state of hypnosis.

You can easily come back to a full wakeful state from a hypnotic state. If you are driving, for example, a beeping horn or a car moving in your direction will jolt you back into full awareness of where you are and what is happening.

Hypnosis works because the mind is divided into two parts called the subconscious and the conscious. The subconscious mind is viewed as the survival, instinctual level of the mind. Everything and every memory are stored in the subconscious mind. The conscious mind, on the other hand, acts as the receiver and processor of information from the outside world. It is the thinking, analyzing, and language processing portion of the mind.

In a hypnotic state, the goal is to slow down the conscious brain waves, allowing the subconscious mind to become open to suggestions. Hypnosis itself, however, is not the same thing as suggestion. Hypnosis is simply the state that promotes the acceptance of suggestions and allows a person to change their thinking, and this change in thinking has been shown to alter the emotional state and affect the sensation of pain.

What Hypnosis Is Not

There are many misconceptions about hypnosis. For example, hypnosis is not:

- A state of sleep.
- A surrender of will to the hypnotist (the person in the hypnotic state maintains control).
- A means by which someone can obtain secrets from the hypnotized person.
- A loss of consciousness.
- A state of mind in which someone can become "stuck" or remain permanently.
- A trance which can only be achieved with unintelligent or gullible people.
- Dangerous.
- A state that can be forced on a person.

Even stage hypnotists do not actually control their hypnotized subjects. These hypnotists perform tests that help them find the most suggestible subjects in the audience. While these people may not remember what happened to them (just as you may fail to consciously remember driving from your office to your home), they would not perform the requests made by the hypnotist unless they wanted to do so on a deep level.

Hypnosis in the Medical/Dental Practice

Every culture since ancient times has used hypnosis to aid in healing. Through the latter part of the 1800s, hypnosis was readily accepted as an adjunct to other medical treatments. When chemical anesthesia became more sophisticated and prominent, however, the use of hypnosis waned. As a result, medical practitioners are often misinformed and needlessly skeptical about what hypnosis is and what it can accomplish.

A certified hypnotist is trained to use the natural state of hypnosis to promote a change in behavior through the use of suggestions in a very specific way. Extensive training is required to learn therapeutic hypnosis for use as a treatment or a therapy. The hypnotist learns how to invoke a hypnotic state of mind so that the subject accepts new ideas (i.e., suggestions) without resistance. Again, however, the subject or the patient must consent to accepting these suggestions and make the decision to let go of resistance.

Pain management is only one way that hypnosis is useful in a medical/dental practice. Historically, hypnosis has been used to successfully treat a wide range of conditions, including anxiety, eating disorders, phobias, fears, and addictive behaviors.

In a January 2000 article in *Jacksonville Medicine* entitled "Homeopathy, Herbs and Hypnosis: Common Practices in Complementary and Alternative Medicine," the authors stated: "Controlled experiments and clinical interventions document the ability of hypnotized individuals to control pain, reduce physiologic arousal in preparation for and during surgery, replace or supplement chemical anesthesia and analgesia and reduce bleeding, swelling, infection, post-operative complications and pain and reduce length of hospital stay. In dentistry, hypnosis is used for psychogenic oral pain, overcoming fear, gagging, tongue thrusting, thumb sucking, flow of saliva and capillary bleeding, bruxism, cooperation with procedures and as an anesthetic in place of chemical anesthesia due to allergies [2]."

Additionally, self-hypnosis techniques can easily be taught to patients so that they can manage pain or deal with other issues, such as habitual behaviors and fears that interfere with treatment protocols.

How Hypnosis Works

The "induction" is the first step in the hypnosis process. There are many types of inductions. In his book, *Essentials of Hypnosis,* Dr. Michael Yapko states, however: "Anything that focuses the person's attention and facilitates feelings of comfort and well-being can be used as an induction [3]." The goal of this vital step in trance initiation is to relax the mind and body, increase mental focus and concentration, and prepare for the acceptance of suggestions.

There is no perfect induction for everyone. The goal is to increase inner sensory awareness while reducing awareness of the outside world, and the way to reach that goal depends upon the individual.

A common induction utilizes a pendulum or a point of focus. A pendulum is simply an object that hangs from something so that it swings freely. You can use a necklace for this, or you can choose some other object as the point of focus.

I generally use five steps when hypnotizing my patients. What follows is a sample:

Step One: Pendulum or Point of Focus and Relaxation Breathing

Remove any mints or candy from your mouth. Sit comfortably, and begin by holding your pendulum or point of focus in your dominant hand in a vertical position between your thumb and forefinger. Center the tip of the pendulum or point of focus one-half inch above the outstretched palm of your non-dominant hand. With your eyes open, place your attention on the tip of the pendulum or the point of focus, and take a breath. Then, count backward out loud as follows: 15, 14, 13, 12, 11, 10, 9, 8, 7, 6, 5, 4, 3, 2, 1. Place the pendulum down and close your eyes, and take a second deep breath.

Imagine golden sun rays of relaxation flowing into your fingertips. As you take a deep breath, feel the tingling sensation of relaxation traveling up your arms to your elbows and all the way up to your shoulders. Then, let it flow into your neck and continue up to the top of your head. Picture the golden sun rays of relaxation spreading from the top of your head ...down your neck ... filling your chest and your heart with healing. Now, down your spinal column, into your stomach and your hips ... down your legs ... all the way to your feet. When you have imagined that the relaxation has reached your toes, wiggle them, and allow yourself to release all of your tension and stress.

Since it is easier to quiet the body than to quiet the mind, deepening of the hypnotic state gives the mind a chance to follow the body into relaxation. The goal of this next step is to bring the patient to a deeper level of trance.

Step Two: Quiet the Mind

Imagine a magical staircase in front of you leading to a private retreat. Authorize yourself to take the first step. You feel excited as you treat yourself with the respect you deserve and start the process of change. On the second step, you feel deeply relaxed. See yourself firmly on the third step. Allow the process of hypnosis to aid you as you continue to move to step 4. On step 5, you feel support from the universe. As you reach step 6 on this magical staircase, you feel yourself moving smoothly and effortlessly into deep hypnosis. Take a moment to breathe in this feeling of well-being as you step onto 7. You feel tranquil and relaxed ... very relaxed. Now, moving onto step 8 ... and as you approach the ninth step, you feel safe and calm, open to helpful suggestions. Step 10 completes your journey as you achieve a receptive state of mind. This is your special time for making a positive change in your life. You are ready.

The next step is to create imagery. This can be achieved with sensory-oriented suggestions for designing a safe place in the mind. This guided visualization is especially effective for patients who have fears or phobias related to treatment. A sample induction of developing a safe place is as follows:

Step Three: Create Imagery

Picture yourself standing at the door of a very safe place. As you open the door, see yourself in this unique, special, wonderful place. Imagine a chair right in front of you. Sit down, and feel the chair supporting you. There is a delicious drink especially for you next to the chair. Pick up the glass, and feel it in your hand. Now, taste the drink, and savor its flavors. Smell the freshness in the air, and listen to the sounds in the background. Take a moment to enjoy the beautiful scenery. This is a special time for transformation. You are allowing yourself to create a healthier body and mind. You are ready to modify your thoughts.

Step Four: Developing Suggestions

Suggestions can be compared to a navigational compass as they direct thoughts that lead the person to achieve their goal. There are many roads to that goal, so it is critical to understand which type of suggestion best suits the individual. For example, if you want the patient to produce more saliva in the mouth, a negative suggestion such as "Do not think of your favorite food" may cause the patient to think of the food and produce the additional saliva.

A positive suggestion, on the other hand, is supportive and encouraging and helps the individual create a visualization of the desired behavior. For example, you might say, "Remember a time when you were very proud of yourself."

The step of developing suggestions needs to be done with a clear vision of the patient and the desired goals. It is critical that the suggestions are acceptable, motivating, and believable to the person receiving them. All suggestions must fit into the individual's belief system and be emotionally acceptable in order to produce a behavioral change.

Step Five: Ending the Session

The final step is to present post-hypnotic suggestions while the patient is in a hypnotic state of mind, which will carry the suggestions into the desired context in the awakened state of mind and facilitate inductions in future hypnotic sessions. These suggestions are designed to reinforce and summarize the newly acquired thinking, integrating the new behaviors so that they become a reality in the future [3].

A sample suggestion might be:

> Day by day, as you move forward, you enjoy each moment. You now feel able to manage your life. You are becoming more and more relaxed and healthy. When you return for the next hypnotic session, you will be able to go into deep hypnosis quickly and easily. You feel ready for the change.

After the post-hypnotic suggestions are completed, the script I generally use to close the hypnosis session is as follows:

> We have now finished our session. You will carry with you all of the new behavior patterns you have learned, as well as a sense of well-being. I will count from 5 to 1, allowing you to slowly return to full alertness, leaving your safe place with the confidence that you will be able to return to it anytime you want. Let's begin: 5 ...beginning to drift back to complete

alertness; 4 ...closer now to complete awareness; 3 ...becoming aware of your surroundings; 2 ... feeling refreshed and rejuvenated; and 1.
   When you feel ready to return to your day, open your eyes, and look forward to positive results from this hypnosis session. You feel refreshed, rejuvenated, and ready.

It is very beneficial to hydrate after a hypnosis session, so I offer a glass of water to help the patient become more alert.

Hypnosis for Eliminating Emotional Roadblocks to Treatment

Fear is a natural instinct that helps us survive in the face of danger. When the body responds, it does not know if the danger is real or imagined. Therefore, the mind can be tricked to react even when a danger does not actually exist, such as when you see a shadow at night and become frightened enough that your heart starts to beat rapidly, you feel faint, and/or you start to sweat. Even when you realize that the danger is not real, it is difficult to turn off the body's reaction.

Medical anxiety is a fear reaction to the unknowns of what might happen during a medical procedure as well as loss of control during the procedure. Anxiety is extremely common, especially in people who are to have a procedure they have never experienced before. Medical anxiety can often be reduced if the patient is given information and knowledge in advance, thus eliminating as many unknowns as possible. It is important to assess the patient's level of anxiety through body language and conversation before beginning the procedure in order to prevent an escalation of anxiety that might have been handled easily if addressed earlier. It is essential to address all questions and concerns and ensure that the patient is ready to begin.

Medical phobia differs from medical anxiety in that it is a fear that develops in people who have never had a bad experience with a procedure. Instead, it is based on indirect experiences such as hearing the negative stories of others or seeing a film with a scene in a doctor's office. "Phobia" is traditionally defined as "an irrational severe fear that leads to avoidance of the feared situation, object, or activity." In most cases, a phobia develops in a person who already suffers from anxiety, and such people avoid care at all costs until the pain becomes overwhelming.

Negative emotions, fears, and stress lead to a feeling of dread and loss of control that cause the body to react with chemical and electrical responses within the nervous system, activating the hypothalamic-pituitary-adrenal axis. Since the brain is the most important part of the nervous system and is made up of tens of billions of nerve cells, every nerve cell produces chemical communicators to correspond with nearby cells.

Cortisol is the hormone that is secreted by the adrenal glands in response to stress, and too much cortisol leads to an increase in blood pressure and blood sugar levels as well as suppression of the immune system. This chemical reaction called the "fight or flight" response is triggered by a feeling of danger created by anxiety. Any contact with the feared stimulus provokes an immediate chemical response, which may take the form of a panic attack.

Benefits of Hypnosis in the Dental Practice

Patients with dental fears, anxieties, or phobias may have a severe physiological fight or flight response while in the dental office. If a patient begins to have a panic attack while in the chair, the medical procedure cannot continue. Certainly, the physical reaction does not calm down immediately and will delay treatment and increase the patient's sensitivity as well as perception of pain and discomfort. Therefore, it is very important to remember that these fears are very real to the patient, and they simply must be addressed before beginning any procedures.

These patients require more time and special considerations and create stress for dental professionals. Often, people who are fearful of dentistry come into the office only when their pain has grown to an emergency state. What happens as a result? They are squeezed in between regular appointments when there is little time for them. Of course, this is the worst possible scenario for treating such a patient. Chances are these patients have neglected their dental health, creating complex dental needs that may be both extensive and expensive.

A 2006 article published in *Contemporary Hypnosis* by the British Society of Experimental and Clinical Hypnosis discusses the use of hypnosis to assist a patient in dealing with her dental phobia. The patient was able to allow the dental procedure to take place, and she learned self-hypnosis techniques that helped her to "feel more confident about accepting future dental treatment without need for pharmacological intervention [4]."

Case Study: Hypnosis for Fear of Treatment

Amanda was a 23-year-old female who complained of head and facial pain which had begun approximately 3 years before. She had been under the care of physicians of various specialties, including acupuncture and manipulative care, and she had also taken prescribed medications. When it became apparent that her pain and dysfunction were not resolving, she was referred to my office by her acupuncturist for further evaluation and treatment. When asked to rate her head pain subjectively using a visual analog scale (VAS), she chose up to a 10 on a scale of 0–10, with 10 designated as the worst pain that she could possibly imagine. She reported that her pain frequently awakened her from sleep and that there were days when it was so severe that she was confined to bed.

Recommended treatment included an intraoral orthopedic appliance, trigger point injections, electrogalvanic stimulation, ultrasound, nutritional recommendations, and neuromuscular reeducation. Amanda needed injections to assist her muscles, ligaments, and tendons to heal, but her fear of injections prevented her past physicians from completing the necessary treatment. Amanda refused injections, saying, "I hate needles, and I faint." She agreed to hypnosis, however, to overcome her needle anxiety.

The goal of hypnosis was to overcome her fear of needles to allow treatment to continue. The hypnosis session started with relaxation breathing and securing an imaginary safe place, followed by the finger focus technique (described later in this chapter) and a post-hypnotic suggestion for continued healing and an easy return to a hypnotic state of mind. Amanda agreed to practice the technique at home through self-hypnosis every day until her next visit.

Amanda did quite well entering a light state of hypnosis on her own. During her next office visit, we reviewed the hypnosis technique and completed the recommended injection treatment. She admits that "hypnosis helped me keep my mind off the needle." Amanda also reports that her pain has reduced and that she is happy with her progress.

Hypnosis for Bruxism

Bruxism involves involuntary or unconscious grinding of the teeth, usually during sleep. This grinding can lead to orofacial pain and residual problems with the teeth and gums. Hypnosis has been found to often be effective in controlling bruxism.

In a study published in the *American Journal of Clinical Hypnosis* in April 1994, a 63-year-old woman, who had suffered from nocturnal bruxism since the age of 3, was treated with hypnosis. Her bruxism had caused facial pain, headaches, and an ulceration on the inside of one of her cheeks.

One suggestion given to the patient during hypnosis included awakening whenever she felt her jaw tighten or her teeth come together, followed by a suggestion that she would easily fall back to sleep. The authors reported, "Three days later the patient reported that she 'had not ground my teeth at all.'" Additionally, the patient reported that her sleep had improved, and the ulceration in her cheek had begun to heal. Even after a 60-month follow-up, the patient reported that she was "cured." Furthermore, the patient's dentist confirmed that the damage to her teeth had ceased [5].

Hypnosis to Relax a Strong Gag Reflex

Another issue that plagues medical professionals, particularly dentists, is the gag reflex, which can interfere with examinations, cleanings, dental X-rays, and treatment. Hypnosis is an effective technique for easing and relaxing strong gag reflexes, and I find that the following suggestion, given after a hypnotic induction, works well.

Place a pen or a pencil in the patient's hand, and say, with confidence:

> "I am going to place this pencil in your hand, and I want you to focus on keeping a steady but gentle pressure on the pencil. Continue to do so, and you will no longer have the desire to gag."

During the treatment, reinforce the suggestion periodically by saying:

> "As you continue to hold the pencil, I want you to visualize, picture, or imagine that as I'm treating you, you will feel calm and relaxed at all times while you focus on the pencil."

Case Study: Hypnosis for Tinnitus

Molly presented in my office, complaining of tinnitus after the completion of dental work on a maxillary tooth which required her mouth to be open for an extended period of time. She described the noise as a "constant smoke alarm going off." When she was asked to rate the noise subjectively using a VAS, she characterized the ringing as up to a 10 on a scale of 0–10, with 10 as the worst noise she could possibly imagine. She said that she could not sleep without the television playing as background noise.

After the first hypnosis session, Molly said that "the sound changed. It wasn't at a 10 anymore. It was reduced to a 7." After four sessions of hypnosis devoted to reducing the ringing in her ears, Molly claims that the tinnitus is only intermittent, and when it occurs, it is only a 3 on the scale. She now maintains that she can sleep without the television.

Hypnosis and Orofacial Pain Management

A continuing study at the Orofacial Pain Clinic in Melbourne, Australia, which is part of The Royal Dental Hospital of Melbourne, was published in the *Australian Dental Journal* in December 1978. The study investigated a total of 200 patients, of which 52 (20 %) received hypnosis treatment involving induction, relaxation, suggestion, and visualization techniques [6].

The author physicians concluded: "It is clear from the types of pain successfully treated that hypnosis is able to reduce or eliminate both 'sensory' and 'suffering' pain. Pain problems, ranging from those of predominately psychogenic origin to those of predominately organic origin, can be managed. Complex interactions of both physical and functional problems are often seen in many instances of chronic orofacial pain. Hypnosis does not merely produce relaxation and relief from anxiety and thus make pain more tolerable; it is capable of reducing pain itself, sometimes completely, sometimes reducing it to acceptable levels."

Case Studies: Hypnosis for Pain Reduction

Anna was a 29-year-old single mother who presented in my office after a car accident that left her with headaches, dizziness, and pain on the right side of her face.

She said, "Medication helps me, but I am afraid to get into a car. And it makes my thinking fuzzy." We scheduled four hypnosis sessions as an adjunct to treatment of the muscles, ligaments, and tendons of the head and neck. The goals of the hypnosis sessions were to reduce fear and anxiety, control pain, reduce medication use, and give her some feeling of control. After the fourth session, she said, "Hypnosis is most definitely a benefit. I had the power to make the pain stop."

A patient named Sally presented in my office for pain in her face resulting from bruxism. Even though this pain had overtaken her life, she was skeptical that her mind was capable of taking her attention away from the grinding that caused her pain. We began the hypnosis session, and as her body began to relax, she also began to cry. Her tears were from relief because she had suddenly and quite easily gained control of her pain. By the next session, Sally's demeanor was very different because she had come to realize that she no longer had to suffer and could exert some control over her painful sensations.

Cautions in Using Hypnosis for Orofacial Pain Management

While hypnosis is a useful addition to treatment of orofacial pain to address the emotional component of the condition, hypnosis can also mask pain. Therefore, when you incorporate hypnosis into a treatment protocol, a clear set of objectives must be identified, and the source of the pain must be accurately diagnosed. Delays in treating the cause could be serious or life threatening, so a prognosis must be achieved before any hypnosis program begins.

All health practitioners should also remain mindful of their limitations when utilizing and teaching hypnosis techniques. A patient might request assistance with a psychological problem, but a medical professional without the proper psychological credentials should never treat such problems. Patients should be referred to specialists for issues that are outside the scope of the treating physician.

Additionally, all medical personnel should obtain a written consent from patients before using any hypnosis techniques. A sample is as follows:

> I am willing to be guided through relaxation, visual imagery, creative visualization, self-hypnosis, and stress reduction processes and techniques for the purpose of self-improvement. I understand that this self-help is not a substitute for medical care. I have been advised to discuss any concerns and undiagnosed pains with any doctor who is taking care of me now or in the future. I understand that despite best efforts, success cannot be guaranteed.
>
> Signed_____

Self-Hypnosis

Self-hypnosis is a technique that patients can use to place themselves in a mentally receptive frame of mind in order to manage their thinking and create new thought patterns. Even though we are not aware of it, we constantly program ourselves using suggestions. Self-hypnosis provides the opportunity to intentionally use the power of suggestion to produce specific benefits.

Using self-hypnosis, an individual can gain control of undesirable behaviors, pain, fears, and destructive emotions and thoughts. The ability to focus on a believable thought or idea that can encourage new behavior is the goal of self-hypnosis, and it is a skill that requires daily practice for maximum benefit.

Self-hypnosis is a perfect tool for use in a medical or a dental practice because it is convenient, easily learned, and of tremendous benefit to the patient with no negative side effects. Patients need to be aware, however, that any new pain that has not yet been diagnosed must be brought to the attention of the treating physician. Pain is a message from the body that requires medical attention and should not be managed solely with hypnotic suggestion.

In an article in the May 2009 issue of *Pain Medicine News,* Mark Jensen, Ph.D., a professor and vice chairman of the Department of Rehabilitation Medicine at the University of Washington, Seattle, reported that the patients who participated in a study of the long-term effects of hypnotic analgesia continued, during the year following their procedures, to use the self-hypnosis skills they had been taught [7].

Self-Hypnosis Induction Techniques

Relaxation Breathing

Whenever we are tense, our breathing becomes shallow. By breathing slowly and with intention, our muscles relax, and we stop chemically triggering excessive amounts of cortisol and adrenaline. This exercise is the first step to prepare for self-hypnosis. It can be prerecorded by you or the patient, or a professionally produced hypnosis CD can be purchased for your patients:

> Take a deep breath, and close your eyes. Imagine that you can breathe in relaxation through your fingertips. Feel the tingling sensation of the relaxation flowing into your fingertips. As you take another deep breath, imagine that this breath carries the relaxation from your fingertips up to your elbows and up your arms. Allow it to flow into your shoulders and up your neck. The relaxation now begins to flow into your head. This feeling of relaxation spreads from the top of your head back down into your neck and your chest, filling your heart with healing breath. The relaxation continues flowing down your spinal column into your stomach and into your hips. Now, it flows down your legs to your knees and all the way down to your feet. Wiggle your toes, and feel the tension leave your body.

Finger Focus Technique

Finger focus is a self-hypnosis technique that I teach many of my patients. This technique allows patients to enter a hypnotic state on their own in order to gain control over negative emotions such as fear.

When the patient places attention on an outstretched index finger, making the finger unbendable, it stops the stream of spiraling negative thoughts by distracting the mind. Concentrating only on the unyielding finger allows for measurable success in thought management, which gives the patient an immediate feeling of control. This technique has helped many of my patients achieve a hypnotic state despite their anxieties. Read the following instructions slowly to your patient:

> Sit comfortably with your lips together, teeth slightly apart, and your shoulders back and down in a relaxed position. Rest your arm on a comfortable surface, if available, and make a fist with one hand, extending your pointer finger horizontally in front of you. Take a deep breath, exhale, and concentrate your full attention on your finger.
>
> Now, tap the length of your finger gently from the knuckle to the tip as you continue to focus your attention on your finger. From the knuckle to the tip, your finger becomes as unbendable as steel. You are empowered by the strength of your thoughts as your finger becomes straighter and unbendable. Try to bend it. Take a deep breath, close your eyes, and let the power from your finger spread throughout your body for healing on all levels.
>
> Now, picture a tube inside of your finger which extends from your knuckle to the fingertip. Allow this tube to collect all of the stress and tension in your body. Your imagination is powerful, and your finger becomes firmer and firmer as your body removes the tension and stress from all parts of your body and collects it in the tube. The relaxation spreads through your body as your finger becomes rock solid and unbendable. Now, imagine that the tube inside your finger is released as you count backward from five to one. Your finger can now bend, and you feel relaxed.

Finger Focus Technique for Children

If you work with children, you can use this same technique with just a few alterations that will help the child to give over to the relaxation of the hypnotic state.

> Would you like to have the power to become a princess or superhero to help you get over your fears? You will learn how to use your mind and your thinking to get this magical power.
>
> In a comfortable position, make a fist with your pointer finger extended. Place your full attention on your pointer finger. Straighten your finger, and imagine in your mind's eye that your finger is becoming unbendable. Tap the length of your finger gently from the knuckle to the tip as you concentrate all of your attention on your finger. From the knuckle to the tip, the finger becomes a magic wand that has special powers. Your finger becomes straighter and unbendable as you receive the magic. Picture yourself in control of this magic power as you focus only on your finger. Try to bend it.
>
> Whenever you need this special power, all you have to do is make your finger unbendable. Take a deep breath, and let the magic power from your finger spread throughout your body. Use this magic power whenever you need it to help you feel better and stronger. When you feel ready to end this session, tap the tip of your finger, and slowly count from one to five, allowing your finger to become flexible again. If your eyes are closed, you will feel happy when you open them.

Intentional Thinking

Our intentions are very powerful. With the intention to relax, resolve fears or phobias, or promote good health, we can often reach goals we never thought possible.

For example, when I was in the throes of my cancer treatment, my mother called me daily to say, "Janet, you need to be positive. Just repeat to yourself, 'I am healthy.'" I did not feel healthy, happy, or positive at all, and I was incapable of faking it. But I realized that I *could* be "intentional" with my thoughts. I no longer tried to control my thinking. Instead, I focused intentionally on one particular thought.

When I put my intention on good health, I ate well, exercised, and got more sleep. So, intentions lead to actions. Positive thinking is fine, but it requires no action. *Intentional* thinking, on the other hand, requires giving direction to thoughts in a meaningful way. Every action begins as a thought; positive intentional thoughts lead to positive actions.

When a patient has mastered the finger focus technique, this self-induced state of hypnosis can be used to plant an intentional thought in the mind.

Ending a Self-Hypnosis Session

In order to end a self-hypnosis session, it helps the patient to make a conscious effort to come back to full waking consciousness. Here are instructions for ending a session:

> Count slowly backward from five to one, imagining yourself refreshed and transformed. When you reach the count of one, open your eyes. In order to get full benefit from this technique, you should drink an eight-ounce glass of water at the end of each session. The water will hydrate you and help you to feel more alert.

Biofeedback

Biofeedback is a beneficial technique in pain management because it gives the patient a chance to control an automatic subconscious activity and bring it into conscious awareness through sensory feedback. Using instruments that measure physical responses, such as heart rate, pain perception, brain waves, breathing, skin temperature, muscle activity, and sweat gland activity, patients can alter individual responses through changes in thinking, breathing, or behavior. As the patient observes the changes as reported by the instrument, he or she can attempt subtle changes to control physiological responses, including pain. For TMJ, for example, biofeedback allows the patient to change activities in the orofacial muscles that are ineffective and which have caused pain or discomfort.

There are a number of different instruments that are used for biofeedback, the most common of which is the electromyograph or EMG. With the EMG, electrodes are placed over a large muscle to measure muscle contractions.

In a study published in *Behavior Therapy* in November 1980, biofeedback proved very effective in controlling the pain of migraine headaches. The authors noted that "temperature biofeedback alone, relaxation training alone, or temperature biofeedback combined with autogenic training were equally effective and significantly superior to medication placebo. For tension headache, the results showed that frontal EMG biofeedback alone, or combined with relaxation training, or relaxation training alone were equally effective and significantly superior to medication placebo or psychological placebo [8]."

In a study published in 1984 in *Behavior Research and Therapy,* 24 patients received EMG biofeedback training for dental fear, and as a result, 21 of the 24 patients "were able to complete dental rehabilitation [9]."

In an article in *The Journal of the American Dental Association* in 2001, author Jeremy Shulman, D.D.S., M.S., discusses the successful use of biofeedback for stopping bruxism in his practice with 90 % of his patients becoming symptom-free after only three or four treatments. It should be noted that a biofeedback splint is utilized to assist patients in becoming aware of and eliminating the bruxing habit. Shulman states: "In my practice, it is highly unusual for a patient to experience no relief, and in such cases, other therapeutic modalities are added. It might be hard to believe that such a simple, quick and noninvasive treatment really works, but once the proper diagnosis is made and major bruxing habits are eliminated, then the dysfunction is controlled and the symptoms disappear [10]."

In a study of eight patients conducted by the Oregon Health Sciences University School of Dentistry published in the *American Journal of Clinical Hypnosis* in 1991, the authors concluded that hypnosis is effective in treating bruxism quickly and that the results last for at least many months. Besides patient reports, the study utilized EMG evaluations to measure masseter muscle activity. These readings confirmed that not only was discomfort and pain reduced, but also the bruxing activity itself was reduced [11].

In a 2008 article in the *Cleveland Clinic Journal of Medicine,* author Karen Olness, M.D., discusses that "hypnosis and biofeedback are cyberphysiologic strategies that enable subjects to develop voluntary control of certain physiologic processes for the purpose of improving health." She also discusses the concurrent use of biofeedback and hypnosis, particularly in treating children, stating: "Adding biofeedback games to self-hypnosis training can make the experience much more interesting for children. Children see evidence on the screen that, by changing their thinking, they have control over a body response such as skin temperature, electrodermal activity, or pulse rate variability. Adults also benefit from the addition of biofeedback to self-hypnosis training. A patient cannot effect a change in a biofeedback response without a change in his or her mental imagery [1]."

Schools and Organizations

Should you wish to become a certified hypnotist, the American Society of Clinical Hypnosis (ASCH) is one of the organizations offering training and credentials. While there are many organizations that provide certification, ASCH is the only one that ensures that its certified members are licensed health care professionals.

Called the ASCH Certification and Approved Consultant Program, it has become a standard for hypnosis practice in the United States. The program requires advanced training in your profession from an accredited institution and licensure in your area of practice and location. It also requires that you have received the minimum required training in clinical hypnosis and that the training has been reviewed by approved peers/consultants.

American Society of Clinical Hypnosis
140 N. Bloomingdale Rd., Bloomingdale, IL 60108-1017
(630/980-4740)

The American Board of Medical Hypnosis (ABMH) provides hypnotist certification for physicians. The American Society of Clinical Hypnosis and the Society of Clinical and Experimental Hypnosis (SCEH) accept certification from ABMH, which is considered to be the highest credential in medical hypnosis, but one of the requirements for certification is at least five years of clinical hypnosis experience in practice.

American Board of Medical Hypnosis
www.abmedhyp.net

Society for Clinical and Experimental Hypnosis
P.O. Box 252, Southborough, MA 01172
(508) 598-5553
www.sceh.us

International Medical and Dental Hypnotherapy Association (IMDHA)
Rural Route #2 Box 2468, Laceyville, PA 18623
(570) 869-1021
www.imdha.com

The Biofeedback Certification Institute of America (BCIA) also requires that those certified in biofeedback are health professionals with appropriate licensure. The organization offers a home study program as well as a list of other training programs that are accepted for certification.

BCIA
10200 W. 44th Avenue, Suite 310 Wheat Ridge, CO 80033-2840
(303) 420-2902
www.bcia.org

Conclusion

Hypnosis, self-hypnosis, and biofeedback are effective techniques to improve both physical and spiritual well-being and give the patient back some control. These techniques have been shown in studies to reduce pain, increase relaxation, decrease or alleviate destructive habitual behaviors, and reduce or alleviate fears and phobias.

When performed by a competent professional, hypnosis and biofeedback are a useful part of a comprehensive treatment plan. Medical/dental practitioners can also teach simple self-hypnosis techniques to their patients which can be used at home for pain control or to manage fears in preparation for procedures. As patients become more adept with self-hypnosis techniques, they can significantly reduce chronic pain, including orofacial pain, and even release lifelong phobias that have prevented them from seeking necessary medical treatment.

A great deal of time and money are spent developing and strengthening our bodies, but training of the mind is often neglected as an integral part of attaining good health. The mind is very powerful. It can affect us not only mentally and emotionally but physically as well.

Acknowledgement None declared.

Conflict of Interest None declared.

References

1. Olness K. Helping children and adults with hypnosis and biofeedback. Cleve Clin J Med. 2008;75(2):S39.
2. Bozzuto A, Bozzuto TM. Homeopathy, herbs and hypnosis: common practices in complementary and alternative medicine. Jacksonville Medicine 2000:17.
3. Yapko MD. Essentials of hypnosis. New York: Brunner-Routledge; 1995.
4. Gow MA. Hypnosis with a 31-year-old female with dental phobia requiring an emergency extraction. Contemp Hypn. 2006;23(2):83–91.
5. LaCrosse MB. Understanding change: five-year follow-up of brief hypnotic treatment of chronic bruxism. Am J Clin Hypn. 1994;36(4):277–9.
6. Gerschman J, Graham Burrows G, Reade P. Hypnotherapy in the treatment of oro-facial pain. Aust Dent J. 1978;43(6):492–6.
7. Kean C. Hypnosis: neglected weapon against chronic pain? Overlooked, inexpensive and safe modality deserves renewed attention, according to experts. Pain Med News. 2009;7:05.
8. Blanchard EB, Andrasik F, Ahles TA, Teders SJ, O'Keefe D. Migraine and tension headache: a meta-analytic review. Behav Ther. 1980;11(5):613–31.
9. Berggren U, Carlsson SG. A psychophysiological therapy for dental fear. Behav Res Ther. 1984;22(5):487–92.
10. Shulman J. Teaching patients how to stop bruxing habits. J Am Dent Assoc. 2001;132:1275–7.
11. Clarke JH, Reynolds PJ. Suggestive hypnotherapy for nocturnal bruxism: a pilot study. Am J Clin Hypn. 1991;33(4):251–3.

Chapter 11
Headaches, Migraine, and Cluster Headache

Ghabi A. Kaspo

Introduction

Primary headaches are those that exist independent from any other medical condition. In contrast, secondary headaches are due to an underlying condition and are classified according to their cause. The primary headaches are discussed in this chapter. The International Headache Society (IHS) [1] classification breaks the primary headache disorders into four categories:

1. Tension-type headache (TTH)
2. Migraine
3. Cluster headache and other trigeminal autonomic cephalalgias
4. Other primary headaches

Tension-Type Headache

Clinical Presentation and Diagnosis

TTH is a common primary headache with tremendous socioeconomic impact. TTHs are so called because they cause a dull aching pain that people describe as a band around their heads radiating to their neck. TTHs are divided into *infrequent episodic, frequent episodic, chronic,* and *probable*. The categories are typically subdivided according to the presence or the absence of pericranial tenderness as assessed by manual palpation.

G.A. Kaspo, D.D.S., D. Orth. (✉)
Clinical instructor of the St. Joseph Hospital-Oakland Dental Residency Program,
Staff at St. Joseph Mercy Hospital of Pontiac and Wayne State University, 3144 John R Road, Suite 100, Troy, MI 48083, USA

Wayne State University - Detroit Medical Centers, 31000 Telegraph Road, Suite 110,
Bingham Farms, MI 48025, USA
e-mail: gakaspodds@gmail.com

TTH is described as a non-pulsating and a dull pain of mild-to-moderate intensity often manifesting as tightness, pressure, or soreness in a "band-like" distribution as if the patient were wearing a hat. The pain location is not specific, though it is often bilateral and may extend into suboccipital and the neck and occasionally the shoulders. Temporalis muscle involvement is most likely present, and mastication may be affected in some patients. TTH is not accompanied by nausea or vomiting, nor is it aggravated by routine physical activity, but it may be associated with sensitivity to light or noises.

The headaches may last from 30 min to 7 days. *Infrequent headaches* occur less than 1 day per month (less than 12 per year) and as *frequent* if they occur on more than 1 day per month but less than 15 days per month for at least 3 months. Chronic TTH evolves from episodic TTH and is diagnosed when headaches occur daily or more often than 15 days per month for at least 3 months. In contrast, if a new-onset daily or unremitting headache with tension-type characteristics develops, the headache is classified as *new daily persistent headache*. Sensitivity to light and/or noises and mild nausea may be present with these headaches. It may be difficult to distinguish between chronic migraine and chronic TTH, and these disorders may be present simultaneously.

Epidemiology

The diagnosis of TTH, a heterogeneous syndrome, is mainly based on the absence of typical features found in other headaches such as migraine. However TTH is the most common headache as about 80 % of the general population suffer from episodic TTHs and 3 % have chronic TTH (CTTH). In a cross-sectional population study of 740 adult subjects, 74 % had experienced TTH within the previous year, while 31 % of the same population had experienced TTH for more than 14 days during the previous year [2]. In another study, a 1-year prevalence rate for TTH in males was 63 % and in females 86 % [3]. The onset of the headaches is usually between 20 and 40 years of age.

Pathogenesis

For many years, TTH was thought to be directly related to muscle tension and was referred to as a *muscle contraction* or a *muscle tension* headache. Muscle tenderness may be present in some individuals; however, increased levels of electromyographic activity are not always associated with the condition [4]. Some studies [5] report that electromyography revealed increased activity in response to emotional stressors in patients compared with controls. It has been suggested, however, that this increase in electromyographic detected activity may not be the cause of the pain but, rather, a response to the pain. Emotional stress, anxiety, and depression seem to have causal relationships with TTHs [6].

A very controversial boundary exists between migraine and TTH. Some experts see these disorders as distinct entities, while others see them as opposite ends of a continuum, varying in severity and features but having a common pathogenesis [7]. At this time, the pathophysiology of TTH remains unclear. The latest theories include peripheral and central sensitization concepts, with a possible role for nitric oxide [8].

Treatment

Establishment of an accurate diagnosis is important before initiation of any treatment.

Simple analgesics are the mainstays for treatment of episodic TTH. Physical therapy and acupuncture are widely used, but the scientific evidence for efficacy is sparse. Nondrug management is crucial. Information, reassurance, and identification of trigger factors may be rewarding. Psychological treatments with scientific evidence for efficacy include relaxation training, EMG biofeedback, and cognitive therapy.

Patients with TTH tend to self-medicate with over-the-counter analgesics, antihistamines, caffeine, and other medications. Rarely do they consult their physician for relief unless the frequency or the severity of these headaches increases. Combination analgesics, triptans, muscle relaxants, and opioids should not be used, and it is crucial to avoid frequent and excessive use of simple analgesics to prevent the development of medication-overuse headache. The efficacy is modest, and treatment is often hampered by side effects. Thus, treatment of frequent TTHs is often difficult, and multidisciplinary treatment strategies can be useful. Since emotional stress plays an important role in TTHs, the patient should be assessed for any significant stressors; when significant stressors are identified, corrective behaviors or, when possible, avoidance should be encouraged. Stress management skills, relaxation training, and biofeedback techniques can be important therapies for TTHs [9], but patients must be willing to take time to work with these therapies. If anxiety disorder and major depression disorder are present, these conditions need to be managed by the proper health care professional.

Pharmacotherapy may be needed, but the patient should be aware of the potential complications. Nonsteroidal anti-inflammatory inhibitors are often effective. Tricyclic antidepressants, such as amitriptyline or nortriptyline, can be helpful in managing frequently occurring TTH but should be taken at bedtime because of their sedative effects.

When masticatory muscle disorders are present in association with TTHs, efforts should be first directed to treating the disorder. A nighttime occlusal appliance for nocturnal bruxism may help a headache that occurs upon awaking. During the day, the patient should practice techniques in cognitive awareness, habit reversal, and self-relaxation to reduce or eliminate tension and clenching or grinding of the teeth.

Often TTH is a heterotopic pain originating in the cervical muscles. When a cervical myofascial pain disorder is present, treatment should be oriented toward resolving this disorder. If myofascial trigger points are the source of headache, the use of postural, stretching, and strengthening exercise programs combined with the use of a vapocoolant spray and/or trigger point injections may be effective [10].

Migraine Headaches

Migraine is a disorder of the trigeminal system. A diagnosis of *migraine* may be confirmed when certain IHS criteria are met after organic disease is excluded: (1) Patients need to have experienced at least five attacks, each lasting 4–72 h; (2) two of the following pain characteristics must be present: unilateral pain, pulsatile quality, moderate-to-severe intensity, and aggravation by routine physical activity; and (3) the attack must be accompanied by nausea (and/or vomiting) or photophobia and phonophobia.

Migraines may occur *with* or *without aura*. *Aura* is the presence of reversible focal neurologic symptoms that gradually develop over 5–20 min and last for no more than 1 h and a simultaneous reduction in regional cerebral blood flow. Aura may also occur in the absence of a typical migraine headache. Patients may experience premonitory symptoms hours to a day or two before a migraine attack (with aura or without aura). These include various combinations of fatigue, difficulty concentrating, neck stiffness, sensitivity to light or sound, nausea, blurred vision, yawning, and pallor. If migraine occurs on more than 15 days per month for at least 3 months in the absence of medication overuse, the migraine is called *chronic*. Chronic migraine typically evolves from episodic migraine over months to years in susceptible individuals. Headaches increase in frequency over time, becoming less intense but more disabling and less responsive to treatment. If migraine headaches last for more than 3 days, it is called *status migrainosus*. Serious complications of migraines are rare and include migrainous stroke, aura, or migraine-triggered seizures and persistent aura [11].

Epidemiology

Estimates of migraine prevalence vary, ranging from 4 % to about 20 % [12–16]. Before puberty onset, migraine is slightly more common in boys, with the highest incidence between 6 and 10 years of age. In females, the incidence is highest between 14 and 19 years of age. In general, females are more commonly affected than males. The prevalence of migraine in the United States is 17–18 % for women and 6 % for men [15–20].

Migraine prevalence is inversely proportional to income, with the low-income group having the highest prevalence. Race and geographic region are also influential factors; the prevalence is highest in North America and Western Europe and among those of European descent [16]. Because the condition usually affects people during their most productive years, migraine is a burden to the patient and society. Not only does migraine affect the patient's quality of life by impairing his or her ability to participate in family, social, and recreational activities, but it also affects society in terms of direct costs (e.g., medical care) and indirect costs (e.g., absenteeism and reduced effectiveness at work).

Pathogenesis

Many mechanisms and theories explaining the causes of migraine have been proposed, although the full picture is still elusive. A strong familial association and the early onset of the disorder suggest a genetic component, which has led some to question whether it is a channelopathy. The trigeminal vascular model by Moskowitz [18] explains that trigeminal activation resulting in the release of neuropeptides produces neurogenic inflammation, increased vascular permeability, and dilation of blood vessels. Other pathophysiologic mechanisms behind migraine have been proposed, such as serotonin, calcitonin gene-related peptide, nitric oxide, dopamine, norepinephrine, glutamate, and other substances [19, 20] as well as mitochondrial [21] dysfunction. It has recently been recognized that central sensitization producing allodynia and hyperalgesia is an important clinical manifestation of migraine [22].

Treatment

Pharmacologic treatment of migraine may be abortive/symptomatic or prophylactic. Patients who experience frequent severe migraines often require both approaches. The choice of treatment should be guided by the frequency of the attacks. Infrequent attacks (two or fewer per week) may be treated with abortive medications [23], and more frequent attacks should be treated with prophylactic medications. If there is a concurrent illness, a single agent should be used to treat both when possible, and agents that might aggravate a comorbid illness should be avoided. Nonpharmacologic methods such as biofeedback, relaxation techniques, acupuncture, and other behavioral interventions can be used as adjunctive therapy [24]. Patient preferences should also be considered.

Several medications have been used for acute migraine treatment, including selective $5\text{-HT}_{1B/D}$ (serotonin) agonists, analgesics, nonsteroidal anti-inflammatory drugs, antiemetics, anxiolytics, ergot alkaloids, steroids, neuroleptics, and narcotics. Drugs with proven statistical and clinical benefit according to the American Academy of Neurology should be given as first-line treatment [23].

When migraine becomes more frequent and the use of acute medications exceeds two to three times per week, preventive medications are used. Preventive treatments include a broad range of medications, most notably antidepressants, anticonvulsants, and beta-blockers [23]. Serotonin antagonists [24, 25], nonsteroidal anti-inflammatory drugs, and calcium channel blockers appear to be less effective [26]. These medications are started at low doses and titrated to the desired effect to minimize the side effects and arrive at the minimal dose needed. In more refractory cases, polypharmacy may be necessary. Botulinum toxin type A is an alternative that continues to be studied [27, 28].

Patients can help themselves, too, by learning to identify and avoid headache triggers. Important triggers are environmental factors, including light, noise, allergens, and barometric changes; behavioral factors, such as missing meals or getting too much or too little sleep; and food/beverage items, such as cured meats, cheese, chocolate, and those containing aspartame, monosodium glutamate, and nitrites.

Cluster Headache

Clinical Presentation and Diagnosis

Cluster headaches are typically side fixed, remaining on the same side of the head for the patient's lifetime. This headache is a throbbing, sharp, or boring pain of severe intensity usually localized to the orbital, supraorbital, and/or temporal region. Only 15 % of patients will experience a side shift between cluster periods. To confirm the diagnosis, patients should have experienced at least five attacks of severe, unilateral, pain lasting from 15 to 180 min if left untreated [1]. The headache also needs to be associated with at least one of the following signs or symptoms: lacrimation, conjunctival injection, rhinorrhea, nasal congestion, forehead and facial sweating, miosis, ptosis, or eyelid edema.

Patients cannot and do not want to remain still during a cluster headache. They typically pace the floor or even bang their heads against the wall to try to alleviate the pain. Cluster headaches are short in duration compared with some of the other primary headache disorders, usually lasting an average of 45 min to 1 h, and patients will frequently have between one and three attacks per day. The headaches have a predilection for the first REM sleep phase, so the patient will awaken with a severe headache 60–90 min after falling asleep. This is an important distinguishing characteristic, as very few other pain problems are known to wake a person from sleep.

Cluster headaches can be of an *episodic* (greater than 1 month of headache-free days per year) or a *chronic* (occurring for more than 1 year without remission or with remissions lasting less than 1 month) subtype. Between 80 and 90 % of cluster patients have the episodic variety. Cluster periods, or the time when patients are experiencing daily cluster headache attacks, usually last between 2 and 12 weeks, and patients can have 1–2 cluster periods per year. It is common for a patient to experience a cluster period at the same time each year. This circadian periodicity suggests a hypothalamic generator for cluster headaches [29].

Epidemiology

Cluster headache was thought to affect primarily men; however, more recent studies have determined the ratio of men to women to be approximately 4:1 [30, 31]. Prevalence estimates vary between 0.09 and 0.32 % [32, 33].

Pathogenesis

The three defining aspects of cluster headache are the trigeminal distribution, periodicity of attacks, and one sided, but the primary mechanism associated with cluster headache is unknown; it is believed to be central. The rhythmic periodicity and the predilection for attacks to occur during sleep have implicated circadian and circannual rhythms, which indicate hypothalamic involvement [29, 34].

Studies have shown a close relationship between cluster headaches and sleep-disordered breathing and sleep apnea [35, 36]. This factor may explain the positive response of cluster headaches to oxygen as well as the relationship between cluster headaches and altitude and sleep apnea [37].

Treatment

The treatment of cluster headache is essentially pharmacologic, with the goal of shortening and alleviating the cluster headache attacks and shortening the cycle of attacks; therefore, like migraine therapy, it can be divided into symptomatic/abortive and prophylactic regimens. Due to the nature of cluster headaches, symptomatic treatment is rapid acting. Agents used are oxygen, serotonin receptor agonists (triptans), and dihydroergotamine. Individual attacks will usually respond to oxygen delivered at 7 L per minute for approximately 15 min. Due to the frequency of headaches, the use of ergotamine preparations is largely limited because of the hypertensive effects of the ergot alkaloid. Also, because of the rapid onset of pain and relatively short duration, oral narcotic analgesics should be limited.

Prophylactic therapies should be initiated as soon as the cycle begins. Verapamil may be used as first-line treatment [38, 40]. Corticosteroids are also very effective but should be used only as initiation therapy for a short period of time [42]. Others, such as lithium carbonate, Divalproex Sodium, and Topiramate, have shown superiority over placebo in several trials [39, 42]. There is insufficient evidence for the use of gabapentin at this time. More controlled trials are needed to establish the appropriate protocol for prophylactic treatment of cluster headaches. The preventive medications are usually continued for 1 month after the last cluster attack and then discontinued until the next cycle begins.

Limited information from small case series is available and indicates varying degrees of success on surgical intervention to treat cluster headaches. The procedures included sphenopalatine ganglion blockade [41, 42], trigeminal rhizotomy [41, 42], microvascular decompression of the trigeminal nerve [42], and gamma knife radiation [43]. More recently, occipital nerve stimulation and deep brain stimulation of the hypothalamic area in patients with intractable chronic cluster headaches have been studied [43–46], and these small case series have yielded promising results. Surgical interventions are reserved for extreme unremitting cases of cluster headache when all medications have failed to provide relief.

Paroxysmal Hemicrania

Paroxysmal hemicrania is a headache with clinical characteristics similar to those of cluster headache, but the headache attacks are shorter lasting (2–30 min), more frequent, and occur more commonly in women [1]. The attacks are also strictly unilateral, predominantly in the periorbital region. The diagnosis is confirmed when the headache is accompanied by at least one of the following signs or symptoms: lacrimation, conjunctival injection, rhinorrhea, nasal congestion, forehead and facial sweating, miosis, ptosis, and eyelid edema. Attacks occurring in periods lasting 7 days to 1 year separated by pain-free periods lasting 1 month or more are classified as *episodic*, and attacks occurring for more than 1 year without remission or with remissions lasting less than 1 month are classified as *chronic*. Unlike with cluster headache, very little is known about the pathophysiologic mechanisms behind paroxysmal hemicrania, but it is thought that disturbances in the hypothalamus play a central role in this entity as well [47].

The disorder is peculiar in that it is 100 % responsive to indomethacin [46–48]. Contrasting reports are available about the efficacy of sumatriptan [49–51]. Topiramate appears to be promising [52].

Acknowledgement None declared.

Conflict of Interest None declared.

References

1. Headache Classification Subcommittee of the International Headache Society. The international classification of headache disorders: 2nd edition. Cephalalgia. 2004;24 Suppl 1:9–160.
2. Rasmussen BK, Jensen R, Olesen J. A population-based analysis of the diagnostic criteria of the International Headache Society. Cephalalgia. 1991;11:129–34.
3. Silberstein S, Mathew N, Saper J, Jenkins S. Botulinum toxin type A as a migraine preventive treatment. For the BOTOX Migraine Clinical Research Group. Headache. 2000;40:445–50.
4. Schoenen J, Gerard P, Pasqua D, VJuprelle M. EMG activity in pericranial muscles during postural variation and mental activity in healthy volunteers and patients with chronic tension type headache. Headache. 1991;31:321–4.
5. Feuerstein M, Bush C, Corbisiero R. Stress and chronic headache: a psychophysiological analysis of mechanisms. J Psychosom Res. 1982;26:167–82.
6. Olesen J. Clinical and pathophysiological observations in migraine and tension-type headache explained by integration of vascular, supraspinal and myofascial inputs. Pain. 1991;46(2):125–32.

7. Jensen R. Mechanisms of tension-type headache. Cephalalgia. 2001;21:786–9.
8. Lipton RB, Stewart WF, Cady R, et al. 2000 Wolfe Award. Sumatriptan for the range of headaches in migraine sufferers: results of the Spectrum Study. Headache. 2000;40(10):783–91.
9. Penzien DB, Rains JC, Lipchik GL, Creer TL. Behavioral interventions for tension-type headache: overview of current therapies and recommendation for a self-management model for chronic headache. Curr Pain Headache Rep. 2004;8:489–99.
10. Graff-Radford SB, Reeves JL, Jaeger B. Management of chronic head and neck pain: effectiveness of altering factors perpetuating myofascial pain. Headache. 1987;27:186–90.
11. Agostoni E, Aliprandi A. The complications of migraine with aura. Neurol Sci. 2006;27 Suppl 2:S91–5.
12. Diamond S, Bigal ME, Silberstein S, Loder E, Reed M, Lipton RB. Patterns of diagnosis and acute and preventive treatment for migraine in the United States: results from the American Migraine Prevalence and Prevention study. Headache. 2007;47:355–63.
13. MacGregor EA, Brandes J, Eikermann A. Migraine prevalence and treatment patterns: the global Migraine and Zolmitriptan Evaluation survey. Headache. 2003;43:19–26.
14. Stewart WF, Lipton RB, Liberman J. Variation in migraine prevalence by race. Neurology. 1996;47:52–9.
15. Lipton RB, Bigal ME, Diamond M, Freitag F, Reed ML, Stewart WF. Migraine prevalence, disease burden, and the need for preventive therapy. Neurology. 2007;68:343–9.
16. Stewart WF, Lipton RB, Celentano DD, Reed ML. Prevalence of migraine headache in the United States. Relation to age, income, race, and other sociodemo-graphic factors. JAMA. 1992;267:64–9.
17. Lipton RB, Diamond S, Reed M, Diamond ML, Stewart WF. Migraine diagnosis and treatment: results from the American Migraine Study II. Headache. 2001;41:638–45.
18. Moskowitz MA. Basic mechanisms in vascular headache. Neurol Clin. 1990;8:801–15.
19. Longoni M, Ferrarese C. Inflammation and excito-toxicity: role in migraine pathogenesis. Neurol Sci. 2006;27 Suppl 2:S107–10.
20. Peroutka SJ. Migraine: a chronic sympathetic nervous system disorder. Headache. 2004;44(1): 53–64.
21. Sparaco M, Feleppa M, Lipton RB, Rapoport AM, Bigal ME. Mitochondrial dysfunction and migraine: evidence and hypotheses. Cephalalgia. 2006;26(4):361–72.
22. Dodick D, Silberstein S. Central sensitization theory of migraine: clinical implications. Headache. 2006;46 Suppl 4:S182–91.
23. Silberstein SD. Practice parameter: evidence-based guidelines for migraine headache (an evidence-based review): report of the Quality Standards Subcommittee of the American Academy of Neurology. Neurology. 2000;55(6):754–62.
24. Holroyd KA, Drew JB. Behavioral approaches to the treatment of migraine. Semin Neurol. 2006;26(2):199–207.
25. Ramadan NM. Current trends in migraine prophylaxis. Headache. 2007;47(1):S52–7.
26. Chronicle E, Mulleners W. Anticonvulsant drugs for migraine prophylaxis. Cochrane Database Syst Rev. 2004;3, CD003226.
27. Conway S, Delplanche C, Crowder J, Rothrock J. Botox therapy for refractory chronic migraine. Headache. 2005;45:355–7.
28. Binder WJ, Brin MF, Blitzer A, Pogoda JM. Botulinum toxin type A (BOTOX) for treatment of migraine. Dis Mon. 2002;48:323–35.
29. May A, Bahra A, Buchel C, Frackowiak RS, Goadsby PJ. Hypothalamic activation in cluster headache attacks. Lancet. 1998;352:275–8.
30. Manzoni GC. Gender ratio of cluster headache over the years: a possible role of changes in lifestyle. Cephalalgia. 1998;18(3):138–42.
31. Bahra A, May A, Goadsby PJ. Cluster headache: a prospective clinical study with diagnostic implications. Neurology. 2002;58(3):354–61.
32. Ekbom K, Ahlborg B, Scheie R. Prevalence of migraine and cluster headache in Swedish men of 18. Headache. 1978;18(1):9–19.

33. Torelli P, Castellini P, Cucurachi L, Devetak M, Lam-bru G, Manzoni GC. Cluster headache prevalence: methodological considerations. A review of the literature. Acta Biomed. 2006; 77(1):4–9.
34. Leone M, Bussone G. A review of hormonal findings in cluster headache. Evidence for hypothalamic involvement. Cephalalgia. 1993;13:309–17.
35. Chervin RD, Zallek SN, Lin X, Hall JM, Sharma N, Hedger KM. Sleep disordered breathing in patients with cluster headache. Neurology. 2000;54:2302–6.
36. Graff-Radford SB, Newman A. Obstructive sleep apnea and cluster headache. Headache. 2004;44:607–10.
37. Kudrow L. A possible role of the carotid body in the pathogenesis of cluster headache. Cephalalgia. 1983;3:241–7.
38. Capobianco DJ, Dodick DW. Diagnosis and treatment of cluster headache. Semin Neurol. 2006;26:242–59.
39. May A, Leone M, Afra J, et al. EFNS guidelines on the treatment of cluster headache and other trigeminal-autonomic cephalalgias. Eur J Neurol. 2006;13:1066–77.
40. Pascual J, Lainez MJ, Dodick D, Hering-Hanit R. Antiepileptic drugs for the treatment of chronic and episodic cluster headache: a review. Headache. 2007;47:S1–89.
41. Taha JM, Tew Jr JM. Long-term results of radiofrequency rhizotomy in the treatment of cluster headache. Headache. 1995;35:193–6.
42. Lovely TJ, Kotsiakis X, Jannetta PJ. The surgical management of chronic cluster headache. Headache. 1998;38:590–4.
43. McClelland 3rd S, Barnett GH, Neyman G, Suh JH. Repeat trigeminal nerve radiosurgery for refractory cluster headache fails to provide long-term pain relief. Headache. 2007;47:298–300.
44. Starr PA, Barbara NM, Raskin NH, Ostrem JL. Chronic stimulation of the posterior hypothalamic region for cluster headache: technique and 1-year results in four patients. J Neurosurg. 2007;106:999–1005.
45. Burns B, Watkins L, Goadsby PJ. Treatment of medically intractable cluster headache by occipital nerve stimulation: long-term follow-up of eight patients. Lancet. 2007;369:1099–106.
46. Leone M, Franzini A, Broggi G, Bussone G. Hypothalamic stimulation for intractable cluster headache: long-term experience. Neurology. 2006;67:150–2.
47. Matharu MS, Goadsby PJ. Functional brain imaging in hemicrania continua: implications for nosology and pathophysiology. Curr Pain Headache Rep. 2005;9:281–8.
48. Antonaci F, Pareja JA, Caminero AB, Sjaastad O. Chronic paroxysmal hemicrania and hemicrania continua. Parenteral indomethacin: the 'indotest'. Headache. 1998;38:122–8.
49. Pascual J, Quijano J. A case of chronic paroxysmal hemicrania responding to subcutaneous sumatriptan. J Neurol Neurosurg Psychiatry. 1998;65:407.
50. Antonaci F, Pareja JA, Caminero AB, Sjaastad O. Chronic paroxysmal hemicrania and hemicrania continua: lack of efficacy of sumatriptan. Headache. 1998;38:197–200.
51. Cohen AS, Goadsby PJ. Paroxysmal hemicrania responding to topiramate. J Neurol Neurosurg Psychiatry. 2007;78:96–7.
52. Cohen AS, Goadsby PJ. Paroxysmal hemicrania responding to topiratnate. J Neurol Neurosurg Psychiatry. 2007;78:96–7.

Chapter 12
Management of Orofacial Neuropathic Pain

Subha Giri

Introduction

The International Association for the Study of Pain (IASP) defined neuropathic pain originally as pain "initiated or caused by a primary lesion or dysfunction in the nervous system" [1]. A revised definition of neuropathic pain as "pain arising as a direct consequence of a lesion or a disease affecting the somatosensory system" was proposed later by the IASP Special Interest Group on neuropathic pain [2]. Neuropathic pain poses a significant challenge to clinicians due to the complexity involved in diagnosing as well as in managing the condition appropriately. For example, a patient with trigeminal neuralgia could undergo multiple dental interventions in an attempt to address the pain, only to have the pain recur elsewhere along the distribution of the trigeminal nerve, thus contributing to frustrations for both the clinician and the patient. Also, in most clinical scenarios, neuropathic pain presents as a chronic pain condition often impacting the quality of life of the patients suffering from it.

A population-based study from Europe estimated the prevalence of chronic pain of neuropathic origin to be at 8 % [3]. In the United States, it is estimated that approximately 3.8 million people have neuropathic pain, including neuropathic back pain [4].

Neuropathic pain is classified based on the location within the nervous system that appears to mediate the pain (peripheral or central), based on the etiology of injury to the nerves (such as trauma, infection, inflammation, neurotoxicity, vitamin deficiency, neuro-degeneration, metabolic disorder) and based on the duration of signs and symptoms of pain presentation, and it is classified as either episodic or continuous pain (Fig. 12.1).

S. Giri, B.D.S., M.S. (✉)
Minnesota Head and Neck Pain Clinic, Twin Cities, MN, USA
e-mail: giri0002@umn.edu

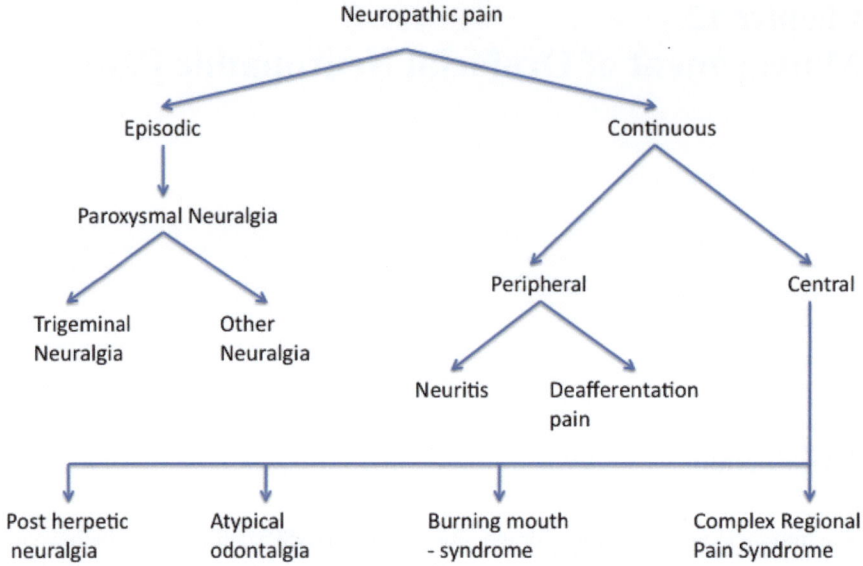

Fig. 12.1 Classification

In this chapter, orofacial neuropathic pain is discussed under the categories of episodic and continuous pain.

Episodic Neuropathic Pain

Episodic neuropathic pain can be further categorized into neurovascular pain and paroxysmal neuralgias. Some examples of episodic neuropathic pain that is neurovascular in presentation include certain primary headache conditions such as migraine, cluster headache, and other autonomic cephalalgia. The discussion on episodic neuropathic pain is limited to paroxysmal neuralgias in this chapter.

Paroxysmal Neuralgia

Clinical Features

Paroxysmal neuralgia is characterized by sudden electric pain that has a bright stimulating quality to it. Other terms used to describe the quality of the pain includes burning, shooting, stabbing, hot, or shocking. Paroxysmal neuralgia occurs predominantly during middle and old age with increase in incidence with age. It is also more prevalent in women than men. The pain presents unilaterally and is felt in the precise anatomic distribution of the involved nerve [5].

The paroxysmal pain is also characterized by the presence of a site in the periphery, in the orofacial region that acts a "trigger zone," which when lightly touched triggers the paroxysmal pain. The location of this "trigger zone" is anatomically related to the location of the pain. Patients are known to report daily activities that trigger the pain including talking, eating, combing hair, or shaving. The paroxysms of pain are frequently followed by a refractory period during which pain cannot be induced by stimulating the "trigger zone." Each paroxysmal episode of pain lasts only for a few seconds at a time. Occasionally patients also report a background dull continuous pain.

Paroxysmal neuralgias are further divided into categories based on location and specific cranial nerve involved in the pain. These include trigeminal neuralgia ("tic douloureux"), glossopharyngeal neuralgia, geniculate neuralgia, superior laryngeal neuralgia, and occipital neuralgia.

Trigeminal neuralgia is the most common clinical diagnosis of all the cranial paroxysmal neuralgia. Due to the anatomic distribution of the trigeminal nerve, trigeminal neuralgia needs to be carefully distinguished from masticatory pain and dental pain. For example, jaw movements such as chewing or swallowing can trigger a paroxysmal episode by stimulating the trigger zone, thus mimicking presentation of masticatory pain. Similarly, triggered pain from occlusal contact on a particular tooth and arresting of the pain from an anesthetic block can indeed pose as a true conflict in accurately diagnosing this pain presentation as trigeminal neuralgia versus odontogenic pain.

Pathophysiology

A complete understanding of the mechanism behind paroxysmal neuralgia is yet to emerge. However, evidence from research has identified demyelination of nerve fibers in the ganglion and/or dorsal horn in neuralgia [6].

Specifically, with respect to trigeminal neuralgia, this can occur by the compression of the trigeminal nerve root as it exited the pons in the posterior cranial fossa, by an aberrant vascular loop of the superior cerebellar artery [7]. Other sources of compression of nerve trunk can be a space-occupying lesion such as a tumor of the cerebropontine angle, arterial aneurysms, or, rarely, malignant tumors that are extramedullary in location. Demyelination of the trigeminal nerve can also be associated with systemic conditions such as multiple sclerosis.

Management

Treatment of paroxysmal neuralgia has to begin with a thorough clinical evaluation of the symptoms and signs followed by appropriate diagnostic testing to exclude systemic conditions as well as space-occupying lesions that may be contributing to the clinical presentation.

(a) Pharmacological treatment strategies

The most effective medication in the management of paroxysmal neuralgia has been carbamazepine. The medication's effectiveness is significant enough that it is prescribed as a diagnostic strategy early in the course of pain management. Carbamazepine, an anticonvulsant, enhances the inactivation of voltage-gated sodium channels, thus delaying the recovery of a nerve that is stimulated by repeat firing of action potentials [8]. This in turn is considered to be its mechanism in reducing spontaneous activity of the involved nerve in neuralgia.

Long-term use of this medication is strongly influenced by its side effect profile including ataxia, drowsiness, fatigue, and, most critically, blood dyscrasias.

Recently, oxcarbazepine has been identified as a comparable medication with respect to its clinical effectiveness against neuralgia, however with less critical side effects. Oxcarbazepine shares the effects of carbamazepine on the voltage-gated sodium channels, thus providing for the same mechanism of action with reduced side effects.

Gabapentin, a calcium channel blocker, has shown clinical effectiveness in the management of neuralgia. Due to its side effects of drowsiness and fatigue, it must be gradually titrated it to an optimal clinical dose. Many of the patients do not reach the target dose of gabapentin related to side effects. A once-daily, gastroretentive formulation of gabapentin, Gralise, was introduced in the marketplace in 2011 with similar efficacy and significantly increased tolerability. Pregabalin is emerging as a noteworthy medication in the management of neuralgic pain although further research in the specific mechanism is warranted [9]. Other medications used independently or concurrent with the medication options listed above include topiramate, baclofen, lamotrigine, amitriptyline, and clonazepam.

Other pharmacological treatment strategies include the use of topical medications on the "trigger zone." Topical application of a long-acting anesthetic agent along with the use of capsaicin has been shown to be clinically effective in providing temporary relief.

(b) Neurosurgical treatment strategies

Patients with paroxysmal neuralgia gain only partial improvement with pharmacological strategies. Approximately 25 % to as high as 50 % of the patients report unsatisfactory results with respect to pain control when medications were used to address their pain. Neurosurgical procedure, albeit being invasive, provides an option for patients suffering from this debilitating condition.

As a better understanding of the demyelination mechanism underlying neuralgia has emerged, peripheral neurosurgical procedures are rarely being attempted to address the pain. Procedures such as peripheral neurectomy and use of neurolytic blocks are now attempted much more cautiously and are usually not one of the primary surgical management options.

Peripheral radiofrequency thermolysis is considered a temporary alternative to the more invasive procedures as it temporarily raises the threshold for pain.

The most common procedures used to treat trigeminal neuralgia are microvascular decompression and rhizotomy. The microvascular decompression is an intracranial procedure in which a physical barrier in the form of a stent or an inflated balloon is placed between the compressed nerve trunk and the offending structure, usually a blood vessel, to prevent compression from contributing to the pain. However, this procedure is a major surgery with all the associated risks, and hence patient selection is a crucial factor in the effectiveness of this procedure [5].

Rhizotomy is a procedure wherein the selected nerve fibers within the ganglion are destroyed by radiofrequency thermocoagulation or with the use of a toxic agent such as glycerol. Rhizotomy is associated with significant risks including but not limited to facial muscle weakness, corneal anesthesia, and loss of facial sensation.

Thus rhizotomy, while offering a neurosurgical option in the management of neuralgia, is also associated with significant risks and like the other procedures outline here needs to be considered carefully.

Continuous Neuropathic Pain

Continuous neuropathic pain conditions are conditions that present as constant, unremitting pain of varying quality and intensity with no period of total remission. These can be further categorized into peripheral, central, and metabolic polyneuropathy. Even though these categories can be recognized with reasonable clarity in the clinical environment, how they vary in their underlying mechanism is yet to be understood.

Pathophysiology

Mechanisms underlying the pathophysiology of continuous neuropathic are both complex and not completely understood. Available evidence indicates the existence of both peripheral and central mechanisms that appear to interact and contribute at different levels to the overall presentation of pain which somewhat explains the varied presentation of continuous neuropathic pain conditions. Peripheral sensitization is a known mechanism wherein the threshold for neural depolarization is lowered by the expression of additional sodium channels and other ion channels in the peripheral nerve following the release of inflammatory mediators associated with nerve injury [10]. Central sensitization is the phenomenon where the depolarization threshold of the spinal tract neurons is lowered following the cascade of events after peripheral sensitization including the release of neurochemicals such as substance P and CGRP [11]. When the processes of peripheral and central sensitization contribute to a prolonged condition, altered gene expression can occur which in turn influences the types and the number of receptors expressed by a nerve. This phenomenon is called neuroplasticity, and once this has occurred, even after the healing of the original source of pain, sustained pain can be present and come to define a continuous neuropathic pain disorder.

Peripheral Continuous Neuropathic Pain

Neuritis Pain

Clinical Features

Neuritis pain occurs after an injury or infection affects the peripheral nerve trunk. This results in a lowered threshold for depolarization in the peripheral nerve and presents as a continuous burning pain along with the other qualities of stimulating sharp or bright pain localized to the site of known inflammation or infection. Neuritis may present with other sensory symptoms of hyperesthesia, hypoesthesia, paresthesia, dysesthesia, or anesthesia. If neuritis is associated with a motor nerve trunk then muscular symptoms of ticks, weakness, or paralysis may co-occur with pain [5]. Some examples of neuritis pain include pain with trigeminal neuritis involving a tooth following surgical procedure, facial nerve neuritis ("Bell's palsy"), glossopharyngeal neuritis, and Tolosa–Hunt syndrome.

Management

Once the etiology of the inflammation or the infection is identified, management of the source of infection is warranted as priority. In the case of a suspected bacterial infection, antibiotics are used. When no identifiable infective source is determined, then administration of steroids should be considered. Early steroid therapy during the course of neuritis appears to reduce the risk of long-term symptoms for the patients.

One of the most significant long-term risks with neuritis pain is associated specifically with herpes zoster infection of the peripheral nerve contributing to post-herpetic neuralgia. Post-herpetic neuralgia is managed with the long-term use of medications such as amitriptyline and gabapentin and occasionally supplemented with the use of topical medications such as capsaicin cream (0.025 or 0.075 %) with long-acting topical anesthetic agents. Neurosurgical procedures outlined earlier have been attempted to treat post-herpetic neuralgia with varying degrees of success.

Deafferentation Pain

Clinical Features

Injury to the peripheral nerve trunk, that is surgical or nonsurgical in nature, can result in the deafferentation of nerve fibers. The resulting pain persists even after considerable regeneration of nerve fibers. Deafferentation pain is characterized by symptoms of paresthesia and dysesthesia, alongside continuous burning pain with a distinct area of numbness or even severe pain.

Management

If the injury to the peripheral nerve trunk is minor, the tissue may gradually heal. But if the injury is significant, microsurgical repair of the injured peripheral nerve trunk has been accomplished successfully. Topical medication, such as capsaicin, can be applied to the painful area along the nerve trunk and has been shown to be effective [12]. A low dose of tricyclic antidepressant such as amitriptyline or the use of gabapentin also shows some clinical effectiveness.

Central Continuous Neuropathic Pain

Atypical Odontalgia

Clinical Features

By definition, known as "toothache of unknown cause," atypical odontalgia, presents as one of the most frustrating conditions for clinicians. Most if not all of the patients presenting this condition have had multiple dental treatments including endodontic procedures, and even extractions, in an attempt to alleviate this pain. Atypical odontalgia has been described as "phantom tooth pain" when it occurs in the site of tooth extraction. This occurs as a continuous dull aching pain that can vary considerably in quality and intensity but is unremitting in nature and can remain unaltered for years with or without intervention.

Management

Owing to the lack of identifiable peripheral etiological factors for this type of continuous neuropathic pain, all treatment strategies attempt to address the probable underlying central mechanism. Tricyclic antidepressants, once again, are proving to be effective in the management of atypical odontalgia.

As adjunctive therapy, gabapentin and pregabalin have also shown improved clinical outcomes.

Summary

Orofacial neuropathic pain conditions, both episodic and continuous, are some of the most frustrating conditions for both the clinicians attempting to manage them and for the patients suffering from them. Management strategies for these pain conditions are primarily medication based. Cognitive Behavioral therapy and, palliative therapy for secondary masticatory pain should be considered concurrently to maximize pain relief for the patients.

Acknowledgement None declared.

Conflict of Interest None declared.

References

1. Merskey H, Bogduk N. Classification of chronic pain. 2nd ed. Seattle, WA: IASP Press; 1994.
2. Treede RD, Jensen TS, Campbell JN, Cruccu G, Dostrovsky JO, Griffin JW, Hansson P, Hughes R, Nurmikko T, Serra J. Redefinition of neuropathic pain and a grading system for clinical use: consensus statement on clinical and research diagnostic criteria. Neurology. 2008;70:1630.
3. Torrance N, Smith BH, Bennett MI, Lee AJ. The epidemiology of chronic pain of predominantly neuropathic origin: results from a general population survey. Pain. 2006;7:281.
4. Bennett GJ. Neuropathic pain: an overview. In: Borsook D, editor. Molecular neurobiology of pain. Seattle, WA: IASP Press; 1997.
5. Okeson JP. Bell's orofacial pains the clinical management of orofacial pain. 6th ed. Carol Stream, IL: Quintessence Publishing Co.; 2005.
6. Kerr FWL. The pathology of trigeminal neuralgia: electron microscopic studies. Arch Neurol. 1966;15:308.
7. Jannetta PJ. Neurocompression in cranial nerve and systemic disease. Ann Surg. 1980;192:518.
8. Backonja MM. Use of anticonvulsants for treatment of neuropathic pain. Neurology. 2002;59:S2.
9. Taylor CP. The biology and pharmacology of a2-d proteins. CNS Drug Rev. 2004;10:183.
10. Devor M. Neuropathic pain and injured nerve: peripheral mechanisms. Br Med Bull. 1991;47:619.
11. Ren K, Dubner R. Central nervous system plasticity and persistent pain. J Orofac Pain. 1999;13:155.
12. Epstein JB, Marcoe JH. Topical application of capsaicin for treatment of oral neuropathic pain and trigeminal neuralgia. Oral Surg Oral Med Oral Pathol. 1994;77:135.

Chapter 13
Preemptive Analgesia and Multimodal Pain Management for Temporomandibular Total Joint Replacement Surgery

Daniel B. Spagnoli and Alan David Kaye

Introduction

Pain is not a single entity but a complex, multifaceted experience. Patients undergoing temporomandibular joint (TMJ) replacement are susceptible to postoperative pain for a number of reasons. Factors that may contribute to significant postoperative pain following TMJ replacement surgery include dense innervation of the face (Fig. 13.1) as represented by Penfield's homunculus on the postcentral gyrus of the cerebral cortex, dense innervation of the TMJ with substance P-secreting neurons, existing preoperative acute and chronic pain, psychological impact of preexisting pain, fear of postoperative pain, neurovascular tissue injuries from previous surgery, preexisting plasticity of the central nervous system, and extent of the surgery [1]. The typical surgical approach for TMJ total joint reconstruction involves a preauricular and a retromandibular approach to place the fossa and condylar components of the joint, respectively. Each of these approaches requires dissection through skin, subcutaneous tissue, fascia, and muscle layers as well as the removal of diseased condyle and a probable release of the temporalis tendon by coronoidectomy. Since many patients undergo simultaneous bilateral joint replacement, the sum of the surgical impact upon the tissues by the four incisions and dissections is considerable (Figs. 13.2 and 13.3). Contemporary patients are well informed and are interested in not only the risks and benefits of their proposed procedure but also the plan for their

---

D.B. Spagnoli, D.D.S., M.S., Ph.D.
Department of Oral & Maxillofacial Surgery, School of Dentistry,
Louisiana State University Health Science Center, New Orleans, LA, USA

A.D. Kaye, M.D., Ph.D. (✉)
Department of Anesthesiology, Louisiana State University School of Medicine,
1542 Tulane Avenue, Room 656, New Orleans, LA, USA

Department of Pharmacology, Louisiana State University Health Science Center,
New Orleans, LA, USA
e-mail: akaye@lsuhsc.edu

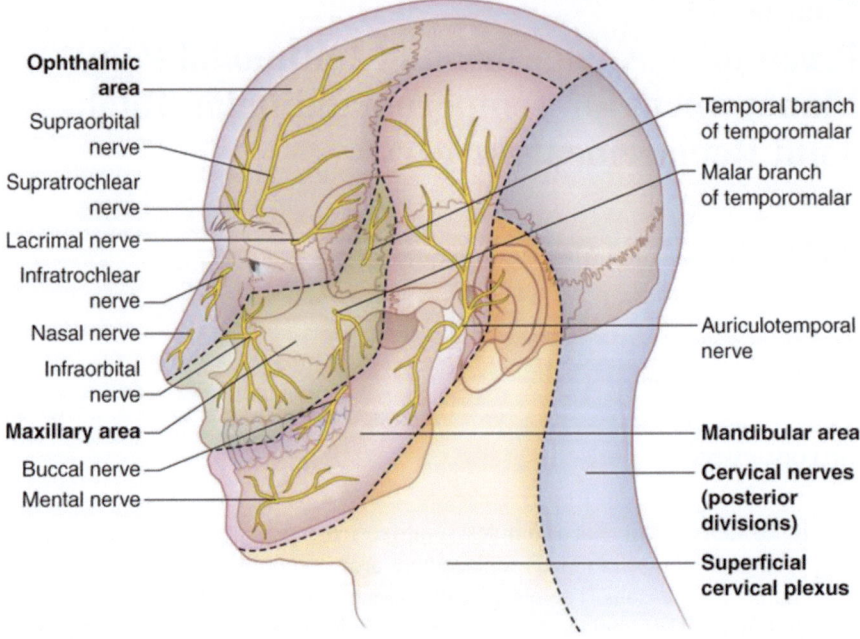

Fig. 13.1 Distribution of sensory nerves to the head (adapted from Gray's Anatomy, 1966)

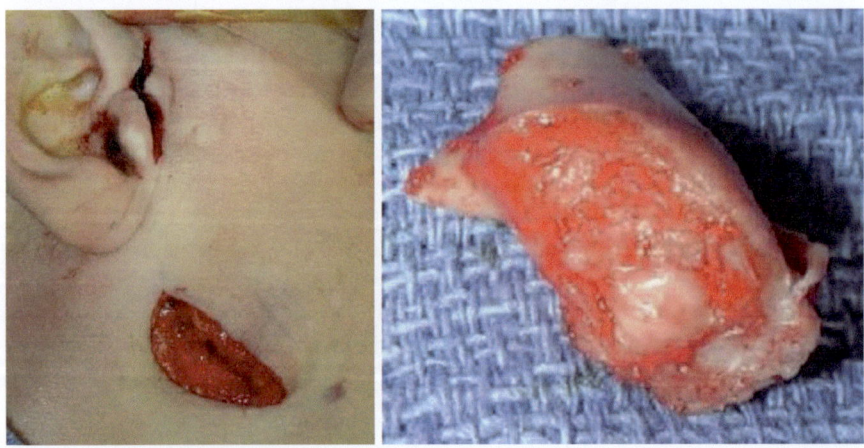

Fig. 13.2 (a) Preauricular and retromandibular incision. (b) Resected condyle with degenerative changes secondary to osteoarthritis

perioperative management, including pain control. The Joint Commission on Accreditation of Health Organizations has published standards for pain assessment and management, and within these guidelines it is stipulated that a surgeon should prospectively include within their operative plan a predesigned strategy for pain management which should be discussed with the patient [2]. Important concepts of

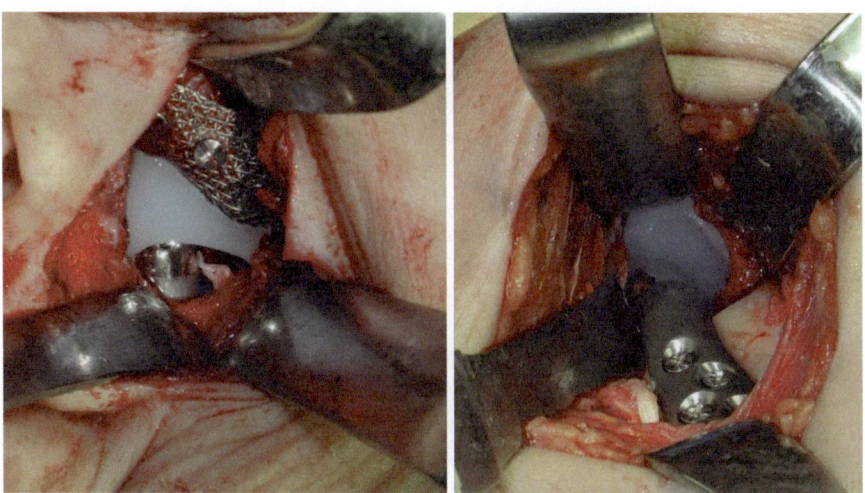

Fig. 13.3 Temporomandibular joint replacement viewed from preauricular and retromandibular perspectives (**a, b**)

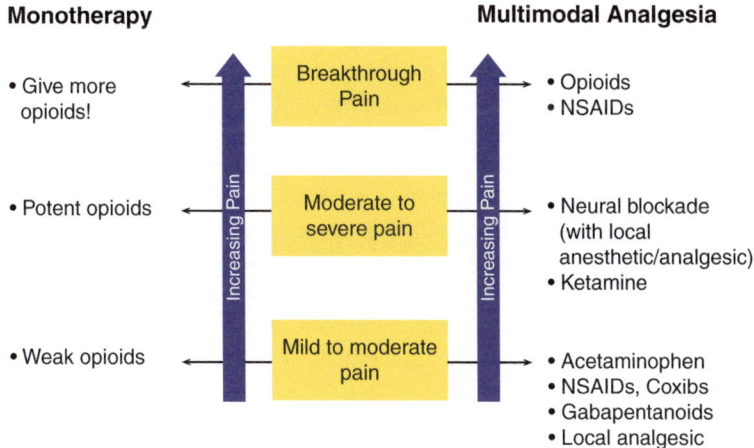

Fig. 13.4 Typical agents employed in multimodal therapy. Exparel™ educational slide set (modified). Modified from Awad IT, et al. Eur J Anaesthesiol 2004;21(5):379–83; Ashburn MA, et al. Anesthesiology 2004;100(6):1573–81; Gottschalk A, Smith D. Am Fam Phys 2001;63:1979–84; Iyengar S, et al. J Pharmacol Exp Ther 2004;311:576–84

acute and chronic pain related to trigeminal nerve pathways have been discussed in previous chapters of this text, although as noted above, patients undergoing joint replacement therapy may have a preexisting chronic pain component that is relative to their outcome. The focus of this chapter is on management of perioperative pain through preemptive analgesia and the neuroprotective benefits of multimodal pain management (Fig. 13.4).

Pain Pathways

Surgical pain is primarily nociceptive and considered to be a complex, unpleasant experience with emotional and cognitive as well as sensory features that occur in response to tissue trauma. Undertreatment of surgical pain can result in many potential consequences, including emotional and physical suffering, sleep disturbance, and respiratory, cardiovascular, gastrointestinal, musculoskeletal, and endocrine side effects, all of which can impact surgical outcome. Some of these include increases in ACTH, cortisol, catecholamines, and interleukin-1 and decreases in insulin levels. Water and sodium retention can occur; decreased mobility which can predispose to pneumonia; muscle splinting, which can result in cough suppression and the potential for hypoxemia and/or pneumonia; sympathetic mediated coronary vasoconstriction, which can result in ischemia, angina, and myocardial infarction; reduced limb blood flow and venous emptying, which can result in venous thrombosis/embolism; decreased intestinal motility and urinary retention; muscle spasm, muscle atrophy, impaired wound healing, and impaired muscle metabolism; increased nerve excitability, which can result in hyperalgesia and allodynia; and finally, sleep deprivation, anxiety, and depression.

Another important consideration regarding pain in the postoperative period is the impact on initiating physical therapy. Patients with uncontrolled pain struggle or avoid participation in physical therapy, whereas those with well-controlled pain, in general, participate in physical therapy within the first 24 h post surgery. To maximize short- and long-term benefits from multimodal pain management the plan should be initiated in the preoperative period continued intraoperatively and extended to the postoperative and post-discharge period.

Preoperative pain assessment for TMJ reconstruction patients is best performed by obtaining a patient history, completing a subjective patient interview, and correlation with a pain questionnaire including visual analog scores. Preexisting pain management should be maximized prior to surgery and may include basic strategies such as splint therapy, physical therapy, acetaminophen, and NSAID therapy, preferably with a COX-2 inhibitor. Acetaminophen, a very weak anti-inflammatory agent, inhibits both COXs by approximately 50 %. The lipoxygenase (LOX) pathway is not affected by any NSAIDs; therefore, leukotriene formation is not suppressed. If patients have chronic pain that requires narcotic therapy, we suggest referral to a pain specialist for management with extended-duration oral or transdermal opiates. If masticatory muscle myalgia and chronic muscle contraction do not respond to other conservative therapies, we recommend Botox treatment of the masseter and temporalis muscles prior to surgery [3]. Our method is the injection of 25 units of Botox A into each temporalis and masseter 2 weeks prior to surgery. Our experience has been that the Botox injections take 7–10 days to become fully therapeutic, and for those patients that require this treatment it not only reduces the muscular component of pain, but it also improves their response to physical therapy.

Table 13.1 Mechanisms of pain perception

Transduction: Activation of peripheral nociceptors.
Transmission: Propagation of action potentials from peripheral nociceptive endings to second-order cells in the dorsal horn.
Central facilitation: Activation of NMDA receptors associated with increased sensitivity and firing frequency of dorsal horn neurons.
Modulation: Different degrees of perception for similar stimuli.

Once a patient's condition is maximized, then they become a candidate for joint replacement therapy. Prior to surgery, we discuss our plan for perioperative and postoperative pain management and physical therapy.

Components of multimodal pain management for the TMJ reconstruction patient must be based upon the classic concept that pain is divided into four overlapping processes (Fig. 13.1, Table 13.1). These processes include *transduction* which is the conversion of energy from thermal, mechanical, or chemical noxious stimuli into nerve impulses by nociceptors; *transmission* of the signal from the nociceptors to the spinal cord and brain; perception or cognition of signals as pain; *modulation* of signals by descending inhibitory and facilitatory input from the cortex that modulates nociceptive transmission at spinal cord or in the case of the trigeminal nerve (Fig. 13.2), projections to the trigeminal brain stem sensory nuclear complex [4]; *central facilitation* involves activation of NMDA receptors associated with increased sensitivity and firing frequency of dorsal horn neurons (Table 13.1).

Surgical pain has incisional and inflammatory components. Incisional pain differs in its mechanism from other inflammatory or neuropathic pain states. Hyperalgesia in the region of the incision is thought to be mediated by sensitization of Aδ-fiber and C-fiber nociceptors and the conversion of mechanically insensitive or silent Aδ nociceptors to mechanically sensitive fibers. C-fiber nociceptors respond to thermal, mechanical, and chemical stimuli, and Aδ-fiber nociceptors respond to mechanical and thermal stimuli. A third system, the Aβ system, is primarily responsible for processing non-noxious mechanical stimuli and serves as a tactile discriminator, but it also plays a role in modulating nociceptive signals that enter the dorsal horn of the spinal cord. These fiber systems are supported by pseudounipolar cell bodies that, along with supportive satellite cells, are located in ganglia of spinal dorsal roots (DRG) and cranial nerves V, VII, IX, and X. The ganglia are located in or adjacent to intervertebral foramina of the spinal column or in or near boney canals and foramina of the skull, respectively. The intervertebral foramina and boney canals allow passage of elements of the peripheral nervous system into and out of the spinal cord and brain stem. The conducting elements of these fiber systems are composed of peripheral axons with free nerve endings or specialized receptor organs that are distributed in peripheral tissues and are contiguous with central elements that terminate either in the dorsal horn of the spinal cord or in the nuclei of the brain stem. They are connected to their respective pseudounipolar perikarya by a T-segment of axonal membrane. No synapses occur between primary afferents in the peripheral ganglia, but the proximity of the neuronal perikarya affords the possibility for electrochemical cross-excitation between neurons to occur.

Transduction, or nociceptor activation, is chemically mediated by substances synthesized or released in association with cellular injury. Arachidonic acid metabolites, leukotrienes, and potassium are released by damaged cells; substance P stimulates nociceptors and also mediates vasodilation and the release of histamine from mast cells; bradykinin is released from plasma secondary to vascular injury, and serotonin is released from platelets. Thus, cellular, vascular, and neuronal injury leads to a rapid nociceptor-mediated pain response which is sustained by inflammatory mediators.

General Concepts and Typical Agents Employed

General Concepts

The rationale behind preemptive analgesia is that injury to nociceptive nerve fibers induces neural and behavioral changes that persist long after the injury has healed or the offending stimulus has been removed. This postinjury pain hypersensitivity can be due to posttraumatic changes in the peripheral and central nervous systems. The noxious stimulus-induced neuroplasticity can be preempted by administration of analgesics or by regional neural blockade.

The concept of multimodal therapies is that a combination of analgesic modalities in perioperative pain management results in better analgesia with a concomitant reduction in adverse effects.

Some established positive consequences of multimodal therapies are allowing for faster recovery and earlier hospital discharge. A component of multimodal therapy is rehabilitation. Generally, there are reduced doses of each analgesic with improved antinociception due to synergistic/additive effects. In theory, there is a reduction of severity of side effects of each drug.

Typical Agents Utilized

- Prophylactic antibiotic
    1. To reduce the risk of a potentially painful infection
- Pretreatment with a COX-2 inhibitor if not contraindicated
    1. To reduce the synthesis of arachidonic acid mediators which are involved with pain and inflammation

- Preoperative dexamethasone
  1. Pain reduction
  2. Nausea reduction
  3. Potent anti-inflammatory
- Balanced anesthesia, including:
- Opioid agent, typically fentanyl, morphine, or hydromorphone, to reduce acute pain. It is well understood that effective acute pain management reduces hospital stays, enhances recovery, and reduces the likelihood of developing chronic pain states.
- Ketamine can reduce opioid tolerance and decrease the dose of opioid required to treat pain. Ketamine possesses N-methyl D-aspartate (NMDA) receptor antagonist effects:
  1. NMDA is a receptor at the spinal cord or the trigeminal brain stem nuclear complex levels that facilitates pain sensitization and opioid tolerance. The NMDA receptor is part of a larger family of glutamate receptors, is involved in the processing of acute and chronic pain, and is an important mediator of rapid excitatory neurotransmission through the nervous system.
  2. Structurally, the NMDA receptor contains four transmembrane channels activated by both glycine and glutamate. Further, the NMDA receptor is divided into three subunits with the NR2B unit most involved in nociception and is thus the area of greatest study for pain-reducing modalities. Ketamine was first developed as an alternative to phencyclidine in 1962, is composed of a racemic mixture of R- and S-enantiomers, and is unique in that it is a central acting anesthetic and analgesic agent. Ketamine is known as the most complete anesthetic agent utilized today underscoring its intense analgesic, sedative, and amnestic properties [6, 7].
  3. Ketamine is ten times more lipid soluble than thiopental, and it is believed to exert its effects via NMDA receptors in addition to central and spinal opioid receptors, serotoninergic receptors, and norepinephrine receptors. Ketamine can be administered via multiple routes as a result of its high lipid solubility. The onset time for the intravenous and intramuscular route is 30–40 s and 3–4 min, respectively [6, 7].
  4. The bioavailability of ketamine after intramuscular administration is approximately 90 %. Ketamine is initially distributed to highly perfused tissues such as the brain, heart, and lung and undergoes redistribution much like thiopental [6, 7].
  5. The drug is metabolized in the liver by the P450 system to norketamine, an active compound which has one-third the activity of the parent drug. Norketamine is then further metabolized into water-soluble metabolites and excreted in the urine displaying an elimination half time of approximately 3 h. Ketamine is the only intravenous anesthetic displaying low protein binding [6, 7].

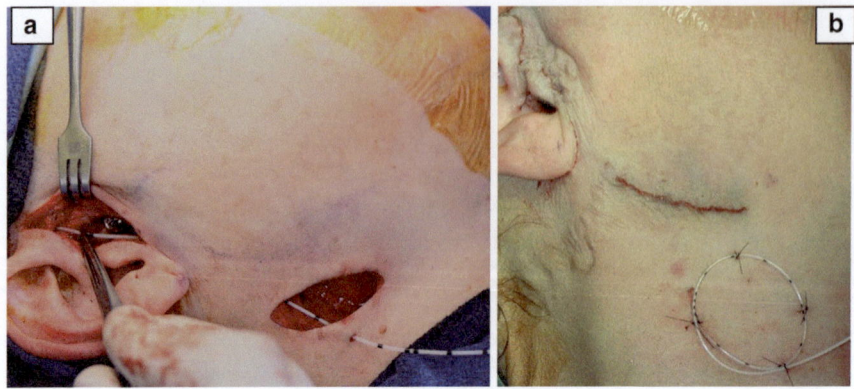

Fig. 13.5 Pain catheter is placed in a subcutaneous plane and sutured at the preauricular and retromandibular level (**a**), skin closure and stabilized catheter (**b**)

- Preemptive and intraoperative local anesthetic auriculotemporal nerve block and incisional infiltration.
    1. Bupivacaine delivered intravascularly can have significant morbidity and mortality.
    2. Ropivacaine has replaced bupivacaine as a preferred long-acting local anesthetic as it is a selective enantiomer that is one carbon different than bupivacaine. If injected intravascularly, it has significantly reduced cardiovascular side effects.
    3. Exparel™ is a novel long-acting liposomal bupivacaine injectable suspension, which was approved by the FDA in October 2011. The technology involves Depofoam, tiny lipid-based particles containing small discrete water-filled chambers dispersed through the lipid matrix. The particles are 10–30 μm in diameter, and the suspension can be injected through a fine needle. Levels persist for approximately 96 h.
- Layered precise dissection that is neurovascular protective.
- Diligent hemostasis to avoid hematoma formation.
- Placement of an I-Flow OnQ pain pump (270 ml, 2 ml/h REF: PM003) which provides local anesthetic 0.2 % ropivacaine for 5 days (Fig. 13.5).
    1. It is important to use the catheter with perforations in the distal portion and not a soaker catheter [8, 9].
    2. This technology allows for an extended delivery mechanism of local anesthesia and longer blockage of pain transmission.
- Continue dexamethasone for three postoperative doses.
- Continue NSAID (ketorolac) or COX-2 and acetaminophen:
    1. Control inflammatory mediators
    2. Control pain mediators

- Morphine, hydromorphone, or fentanyl (rarely utilized) patient-controlled analgesia (PCA) for opiate-dependent patients and for breakthrough acute pain.
  1. Typical PCA protocol; we prefer to use hydromorphone.
  2. Hydromorphone is five times as potent as morphine, has no metabolites, and possesses less side effects. Hydromorphone is very water soluble allowing for a very concentrated solutions.
  3. Morphine is glucuronidated to morphine-3-glucuronide (80 %) and morphine-6-glucuronide (10 %) and normorphine. Morphine-6-glucuronide is an active metabolite. Morphine-3-glucuronide is hyperalgesic.
  4. The continuous PCA setting is rarely utilized, with the exception of opiate-dependent patients.
  5. Typical bolus dose:

  Morphine: 1 mg (0.5–2 mg)
  Hydromorphone: 0.2 mg (0.1–0.4 mg)
  Lockout: 6 min (5–12 min)
  Hourly limit: Ten doses (5–10)
  Basal rate: 0 mg/h (0–2 mg/h)
  Clinician (nurse-activated) dose

- Continuous ice
  1. Decreased vasodilation and swelling and decreased pain transmission.
- Range of motion (ROM) exercise with Therabite or a similar device
  1. Typically start in the morning on postoperative day one.
  2. Improved distribution of medication to the tissue.
  3. Faster return of range of motion.
- Continue ice on discharge.
- Continue COX-2 and acetaminophen or oral hydrocodone.
- Continue ROM exercise.
- Formal physical therapy within 7 days.

In summary, preemptive analgesia and a multimodal approach to pain management, such as described in this brief chapter, can significantly reduce pain and the need to maximize the dose of a single therapy. One of the overlying concepts of multimodal therapy is a lower amount of any one given agent, in combination with others, which might impact pain through a different mechanism or process. Another overlying concept of multimodal therapy is that smaller amounts of each agent can reduce the risks of side effects from larger doses of any one particle drug (e.g., respiratory and/or central nervous system depression with large amounts of opiate). Poorly treated postoperative pain can lead to the chronic pain states which are much more difficult to suppress [10, 11].

In conclusion, multimodal therapy for TMJ replacement leads to improved patient satisfaction, reduced pain-related morbidities, reduced opiate side effects, earlier discharge, improved participation in physical therapy, and in many instances a reduction in total cost. The development of new therapies such as extended-release bupivacaine (Exparel™) may eventually further simplify the administration of multimodal pain therapy, and the use of other analgesics such as gabapentin (a calcium channel blocker, now available in a gastroretentive formation that reduces overall side effects significantly (e.g., Gralise)) may eventually reduce or potentially replace opiates as the mainstay of postoperative pain management.

Acknowledgement None declared.

Conflict of Interest None declared.

Disclosure Statement The authors have no relationships with pharmaceutical companies or products to disclose, nor do they discuss off-label or investigative products in this chapter.

References

1. Asaki S. Sensory innervation of temporomandibular joint disk. J Orthopedic Surg. 2006;14(1):3–8.
2. Joint Commission on Accreditation of Healthcare Organizations. Pain management standards. Effective January 1, 2001. Available at: http://www.jcaho.org/standard/pain_hap.html.
3. Inde SK, Konstantinovic VS. The therapeutic use of botulism toxin in cervical and maxillofacial conditions: an evidence based review. Oral Surg Oral Med Oral Path Oral Radiol Endod. 2007;104(2):e1–11.
4. Sessle B. Acute and chronic craniofacial pain: brainstem mechanisms of nociceptive transmission and neuroplasticity and their clinical correlates. Crit Rev Oral Biol Med. 2000;1(1):57–91.
5. Elia N, Tramer M. Ketamine and postoperative pain – a quantitative systematic review of randomized trials. Pain. 2005;2005(113):61–70.
6. Nadjat-Haiem C. NMDA antagonists. In: The essence of analgesia and analgesics. New York: Cambridge University Press; 2011. p. 316–27.
7. Messieha Z, Cruz-Gonzalez W, Hakim MI. Retrospective outcomes evaluation of 100 parenteral moderate and deep sedations conducted in a general practice dental residency. Anesth Prog. 2008;55(4):116–20.
8. Dhasmana S, Singh V. Continuous ropivacaine infusion vs transdermal fentanyl for providing postoperative analgesia following temporomandibular joint interpositional gap arthroplasty. Natl J Maxillofac Surg. 2010;1(2):112–6.
9. Chelly JE, Ghisi D, Fanelli A. Continuous peripheral nerve blocks in acute pain management. Br J Anesth. 2010;105(51):i86–96.
10. Warfield CA, Kahn CH. Anesthesiology. 1995;83(5):1090–4.
11. Beauregard L, Pomp A, Choiniere M. Can J Anesth. 1998;45(4):304–11.

Chapter 14
Masticatory Myofascial Pain

Subha Giri

Introduction

Masticatory myalgia is characterized by pain and dysfunction arising from pathologic and functional processes in the masticatory muscles. There are a number of distinct muscle disorder subtypes in the masticatory system including myofascial pain, myositis, muscle spasm, and muscle contracture [1]. Among these, myofascial pain is expressed as the most common muscle pain disorder [2]. It presents as an acute to chronic condition that includes regional pain associated with tender areas called *trigger points*, which are expressed in taut bands of skeletal muscles. Although the pain is most often expressed in the region over the trigger point, pain can be referred to areas distant from the trigger points such as temporalis muscle trigger point referring to the frontal area and masseter muscle trigger point referring to the ear and/or the posterior teeth. Reproducible duplication of pain complaints with specific palpation of the tender area is often diagnostic. Pain disorders that are muscular in origin are the most common cause of chronic pain in the head and neck region affecting about 50 % of a chronic head and neck pain population [3]. It is also a common cause of pain in the general population with 20–50 % having the disorder with about 6 % having symptoms severe enough to warrant treatment [4, 5].

S. Giri, B.D.S., M.S. (✉)
Minnesota Head and Neck Pain Clinic, Twin Cities, MN, USA
e-mail: giri0002@umn.edu

Clinical Presentation

The major characteristics of masticatory myalgia include pain, muscle tenderness, limited range of motion, other symptoms such as fatigability, stiffness, and subjective weakness. Comorbid conditions and complicating factors are also common and discussed.

Pain

The common sites of pain in the masticatory system include jaw, facial, temple, frontal or occipital, pre-auricular, ear, and neck. The pain is often a constant steady dull ache that fluctuates in intensity and can be acute to chronic. The duration may vary from hours to days.

Muscle Tenderness

With myofascial pain, the tenderness is deep and localized (2–5 mm) in a taut band of skeletal muscle called *trigger points* [6]. Myofascial trigger points are very common and may be active or latent. A trigger point that is tender to palpation with a single finger and deep pressure and palpation of which results in pain that is continuous at the site of the pain is called an active trigger point. A trigger point which is only tender to single-finger palpation but palpation of which does not result in continuous pain is called a latent trigger point. By definition, when an active trigger point is palpated it must elicit either aggravation or alleviation of pain at the site of pain. Such a site, a specific region of the body, where the phenomena caused by trigger points are observed is called the "zone of reference." When a trigger point is palpated, the referral pattern of pain is usually reproducible across patients. Hence, this predictable referral pattern of pain is clinically used to identify the specific trigger point that is contributing to the patient's symptoms.

Limited Range of Motion

With myofascial pain, limitation in the range of motion may be slight (10–20 %) and unrelated to joint restriction. This mild restriction in the range of motion can result in the aggravation of the existing trigger point and can contribute to the development of new trigger points in the region. The new trigger points along with the existing trigger point can influence the presentation of pain, now contributing to the zone of reference.

Other Symptoms

The patient may present other signs and symptoms including increased fatigability; stiffness; subjective weakness; pain with movement; otological symptoms including dizziness, tinnitus, and plugged ears; paresthesias including numb feelings; decreased sensation and tingling; and dermatographia including increased redness of the skin upon palpation or rolling. The restriction in the range of motion of the affected muscles is associated with the subjective symptoms of stiffness or tightness in the muscle. The patient experiences pain with function and usually guards the muscle from stretching. Prolonged periods of muscle guarding can contribute to poor posture.

Comorbid Conditions and Contributing Factors

There are many comorbid conditions to masticatory myofascial pain that reflect both common etiologic factors and mechanisms of pain. Fibromyalgia is one such condition with widespread muscle pain presentation. As many as 16 locations of the "tender points" associated with fibromyalgia overlap with the location of myofascial trigger points [7]. Hence, fibromyalgia needs to be differentiated from myofascial pain in order to treat these conditions effectively. Fibromyalgia is associated with other clinical findings such as sleep disorder, fatigue, and morning stiffness, while myofascial pain is associated with localized contributing factors such as parafunctional habits and postural factors. Clinically, patients with fibromyalgia are tender in widespread areas of the body, while patients with myofascial pain report tenderness restricted to taut bands of muscular trigger points and along the referral pattern for those trigger points.

Other comorbid conditions that have often been cited to accompany a myogenous disorder like myofascial pain are joint disk displacement and osteoarthritis, malocclusion and functional occlusal dysfunction, connective tissue diseases, neuropathic pain disorders, migraine and tension-type headaches, gastrointestinal disorders, and hypothyroidism. The underlying mechanisms for the coexistence of these comorbid conditions are not yet understood. Common underlying central and peripheral mechanisms and etiologies may play a role.

Furthermore, many associated behavioral and psychosocial factors can accompany the chronic pain associated with a myogenous disorder like myofascial pain. Some examples of behavioral contributing factors are oral parafunctional habits, maladaptive postural habits, and habitual muscle guarding. Some examples of psychological contributing factors are anxiety and depression.

Etiology and Epidemiology

Etiologic Factors

Myofascial pain can be induced by direct or indirect macro-trauma to the muscle or by activities that produce repetitive strain to the muscle [8]. Macro-trauma to the muscle can be from a direct blow to the jaw or from opening the mouth too wide or for too long a period during activities such as dental visits, eating, yawning, and sexual activity. Indirect macro-trauma to the muscle can result from a whiplash type of injury. Local infection and trauma may result in myositis and lead to muscle contracture if not resolved. Occupational and repetitive strain injury can also result in myofascial pain and muscle spasm. Sleep disturbance and nocturnal habits can also contribute to myofascial pain.

Oral parafunctional habits such as teeth clenching, jaw thrust, gum chewing, and jaw tensing and additionally postural factors such as forward head posture, increased spinal curvature, malocclusion, and poor resting posture of the tongue have also been known to contribute to myofascial pain. Psychosocial stressors such as relationship conflicts, monetary problems, and poor pacing skills can play an indirect role.

Pathophysiology and Mechanisms

Since there are no specific anatomical changes in myofascial pain, there are no conclusive mechanisms identified in non-traumatic situations. Thus, there are several processes that may explain the development and persistence of masticatory myofascial pain [8].

Repetitive Strain Hypotheses

According to this hypothesis, repetitive strain from oral parafunctional habits can contribute to increase in oxidative metabolism in localized regions within the muscle which in turn can result in decreased levels of ATP, ADP, and phosphoryl creatinine and abnormal tissue oxygenation, thus depleting the muscular energy. In such a localized region of muscle where the energy is depleted, the nociceptive afferent nerve endings in muscles (type III and type IV), when exposed to substances such as prostaglandins and histamine, can result in pain and tenderness to palpation of the muscle.

Neurophysiological Hypothesis

Tonic muscular hyperactivity may be a normal protective adaptation to pain instead of its cause. As per this hypothesis, phasic modulation of excitatory and inhibitory interneurons supplied by high-threshold sensory afferents may be involved.

Central Hypotheses

Convergence of multiple afferent inputs from the muscle and other visceral and somatic structures in the dorsal horn (Lamina I or V) of the spinal cord can result in perception of local and referred pain [9].

Central Biasing Mechanism

Multiple peripheral and central factors may inhibit or facilitate central input through modulatory influence of the brain stem. This may explain the diverse factors that can exacerbate or alleviate the pain such as stress, repetitive strain, poor posture, relaxation, medications, temperature change, massage, local anesthetic injections, and electrical stimulation.

Diagnostic Tests

Radiographic assessment of the region of muscle pain appears within normal range in patient with myofascial pain. Laboratory investigations of blood and urine samples also are normal unless the patient has concurrent systemic diagnoses that could influence those studies. Trigger point injections with local anesthetic agents can be used as a diagnostic test to identify active trigger points. When a local anesthetic agent is injected into the active trigger point, it results in alleviation of the tenderness and referred pain, either partially or completely. While routine clinical electromyographic (EMG) studies appear abnormal in muscle spasm only, occasionally in myofascial pain, electromyography of the localized region of muscle pain may reveal altered muscle tone. Pain questionnaires such as the Chronic Pain Battery and TMJ Scale may identify contributing factors including emotional issues, somatization, secondary gain, and disability.

Treatment

Simple to Complex

Treatment of myofascial pain can range from simple to comprehensive treatment programs, depending upon the clinical severity of the condition. A wide array of treatment options are available to address myofascial pain ranging from home care exercises and postural correction to trigger point injections, spray and stretch with vapocoolant sprays, and transcutaneous electrical nerve stimulations (TENS).

Medications including tricyclic antidepressants and muscle relaxant also are available as adjunct therapeutic agents. Cognitive behavioral therapy (CBT) along with biofeedback also complements the other treatment options mentioned above. In order to achieve optimal outcomes with the treatment approaches, it is imperative to address the symptoms only after assessing the patients' need and defining it in terms of the clinical severity of the condition being simple to complex. Prognosis and outcomes to treatment approaches are influenced by the identification and management of the variety of contributing factors affecting the clinical severity of the condition.

When the clinical severity of the condition is mild to moderate, with pain being limited to a localized region of the body, along with limited contributing factors and/or comorbidities, the treatment approach can be tailored to be conservative and outcomes tend to be predictable with good prognosis. When the clinical severity of the condition is moderate to severe, with pain diffused in widespread regions of the body, with multiple contributing factors and/or comorbidities, a multidisciplinary team with a comprehensive treatment program is warranted in order to optimally manage the symptoms. Treatment goals also need to be defined for both simple and complex clinical conditions. The short-term goals would be to improve muscle tone, establish pain-free muscle function, and restore normal range of motion. The long-term goals would be to maintain muscle tone and function, using daily maintenance exercise routines and postural awareness and correction on a day-to-day basis. It is imperative to engage patients and have them communicate their personal goals, as it pertains to clinical care, with the assigned multidisciplinary treatment team so as to best position them to gain independence in managing the condition.

Addressing the contributing factors is of utmost importance as this influences the long-term outcome with the treatment approaches. Contributing factors are usually integrated to the patient's lifestyle and environment and hence are difficult to address without the patient's compliance with the multidisciplinary treatment approach. For example, patients need to be compliant with guidelines for postural correction, parafunctional habit reversal techniques, biofeedback, and stress management approaches, all of which integrate to form a comprehensive treatment program.

Treatment approaches directed at the site of muscle pain including physical therapy exercises and modalities, home care strategies, trigger point injections, and use of TENS help address the peripheral component of myofascial pain. Treatment approaches directed at addressing the contributing factors, stress, comorbidities, and systemic health factors help address the central modulating components of the condition.

Self-Care

Most acute symptoms are self-limited and resolve with minimal intervention. Initial treatment should be a self-care program (Table 14.1) to reduce repetitive strain of the masticatory system and encourage relaxation and healing of the muscles. This

Table 14.1 Palliative self-care program for acute episodes of masticatory myofascial pain

1. Eat a soft diet and avoid caffeine.
2. Keep your tongue up gently resting on the palate with your teeth apart and jaw relaxed.
3. Chew on both sides at the same time or alternate sides to minimize strain to muscles.
4. Avoid oral parafunctional habits such as clenching and grinding the teeth, jaw tensing, or gum chewing.
5. Avoid excessive or prolonged opening of mouth.
6. Avoid sleeping on your stomach to minimize strain to the jaw during sleep.
7. Use over-the-counter analgesics or nonsteroidal anti-inflammatory drugs as needed for pain.
8. Apply heat or ice over the tender muscles.

strategy includes jaw range of motion exercises, oral habit change, and protective gentle use of the jaw. Most patients respond well to self-care in 4–6 weeks; if not, further assessment and treatments are indicated.

Orthopedic Intraoral Splints

Intraoral splints can encourage relaxation of the muscles, alter muscular recruitment patterns, and reduce oral habits. Stabilization splints allow passive protection of the jaw and reduction of oral habits due to the flat passive occlusal surface on mandibular or maxillary teeth. Mandibular splints can be smaller and are associated with higher patient satisfaction in some cases. It should be adjusted to achieve mutually protected occlusion with bilateral balanced contact on all posterior teeth with the condyles in their most seated positions, with anterior guidance (lateral and protrusive) provided by the cuspids and/or incisors.

Anterior repositioning splints can be efficacious for concomitant joint problems with intermittent jaw locking with limited range of motion, especially upon awakening, and are recommended for short-term, part-time use, primarily during sleep, because they can cause occlusal changes if worn continuously or chronically. Partial coverage splints may cause occlusal changes in some patients. Splints should cover all of the mandibular or the maxillary teeth to prevent movement of uncovered teeth, with malocclusion.

Cognitive Behavioral Therapy

CBT approaches can help change maladaptive habits and behaviors that contribute to myofascial pain such as jaw tensing, teeth clenching, and teeth grinding. Although many simple habits are easily abandoned when the patient becomes aware of them, changing persistent habits requires a structured program that is facilitated by a clinician trained in behavioral strategies. Habits do not change themselves. Patients are responsible for initiating and maintaining behavior changes.

Habit reversal can be accomplished by (1) becoming more aware of the habit, (2) knowing how to correct it (i.e., what to do with the teeth and tongue), and (3) knowing why to correct it. Patient's commitment to conscientious self-monitoring and focus upon the goal are required for habit reversal to be accomplished. Patients should attempt to correcting the habit during the day and then help reduce it at night. Supplementing with additional behavioral strategies such as biofeedback, meditation, stress management, or relaxation techniques can also help. It is also important to address poor pacing or hurrying related to a day overloaded with commitments and depression, anxiety, sleep disorders, and emotional problems through behavioral and psychological therapy and/or medications.

Physical Therapy Exercises

The most useful exercise techniques for muscle rehabilitation include muscle-stretching, posture, and strengthening exercises [10–13]. A home exercise program directed at reducing pain with muscle function usually involves passive and active muscle stretching. Postural awareness and training are used to address the risk of muscle re-injury. Additionally, strengthening exercises influence the general conditioning of the muscle, thus becoming a component of the long-term maintenance strategy.

At the time of clinical evaluation, the range of motion and functional health of the muscle are baselined. With respect to myofascial pain of the head and neck, both oro-mandibular range of motion and cervical range of motion are evaluated. Myofascial pain of the masticatory muscles, when involving the elevator muscles of the mandible (temporalis, masseter, and medial pterygoid), can result in reduced oro-mandibular range of motion. The oro-mandibular range of motion is measured inter-incisally and ranges between 42 and 60 mm in normal individuals and can be as limited as 10–20 mm in the presence of muscular contracture. While assessing for myofascial pain, other causes of restricted oro-mandibular range of motion including temporomandibular disc disorders need to evaluated to establish or exclude comorbidities. Once myofascial pain is established as the etiology for the restricted oro-mandibular range of motion, stretching exercises, both passive and active, are used to improve it. Patients are always guided with stretching exercises with increasing increments of exercise intensity to avoid re-injury risks.

Physical therapy exercises can also influence the resting posture of the masticatory and cervical musculature. During initial evaluation the resting cervical posture and oro-mandibular posture are noted, and the postural errors are brought to the attention of the patient. Corrective postural guidance with exercises is provided to the patient to establish the most-balanced rest posture. The correct oro-mandibular rest posture is achieved when the tip of the tongue gently rests on the roof of the mouth with the teeth being apart and jaw relaxed. The optimal cervical rest posture is achieved with the chin tucked in and the vertex of the head being held upright. With this, the shoulders relax and sit back instead of being rotated forward. Postural errors with sitting, standing, and walking all need to be evaluated, and correctional postures need to be provided for optimal treatment outcomes.

Physical Therapy Modalities

Therapeutic modalities for myofascial pain include thermal modalities, ultrasound, massage, and electrical stimulation. Use of moist heat and ice pack provides for counterstimulation and changing the temperature of the localized region of pain. Mechanical stimulation of the region with massage and ultrasound helps to reduce tenderness in the muscle, as they improve circulation in the region of pain. Electrical stimulation, TENS, and electro-acupuncture techniques are modalities that address the tenderness and pain by directly stimulating the trigger point. The *spray and stretch* technique with the use of a vapocoolant agent such as fluorimethane or ethyl chloride is also used as a modality that improves the effectiveness of the muscle stretch that accompanies the cooling effect of the agents used. In this technique a fine stream of the vapocoolant is sprayed towards the skin over the trigger point at an acute angle of approximately 30°, and as the stream of vapocoolant is sprayed in a sweeping motion, the patient is guided to do a passive stretching exercise of the muscle to complement the gentle repetitive sweeps of the spray.

Trigger Point Dry Needling and Trigger Point Injections

Generally, the placement of a local anesthetic agent in an active trigger point is called as a *trigger point injection*. Patients receiving trigger point injections may notice improvement in symptoms, that could last from few hours to few days and even few months with a single delivery of the local anesthetic. Other agents that have been used with the trigger point injection include dexamethasone and saline. The effectiveness of the trigger point injection is influenced by accurately locating the active trigger point with the needle. When accurately located, the needling of the trigger point elicits a twitch response in the taut band. Trigger point dry needling is a technique where the accurately placed needle can be manipulated in itself to produce the effect of reduced tenderness and pain in the localized region of pain. For the trigger point injection with a local anesthetic, the commonly used anesthetics are bupivacaine hydrochloride (Marcaine) and carbocaine (mepivacaine).

Pharmacotherapy

Pharmacotherapy is a useful adjunct to initial treatment of muscle pain. The most commonly used medications for pain are classified as nonnarcotic analgesics (nonsteroidal anti-inflammatories), narcotic analgesics, muscle relaxants, tranquilizers, nonsteroidal sedatives, and antidepressants. Analgesics are used for addressing pain, muscle relaxants and tranquilizers for anxiety, fear, and muscle tension; sedatives for enhancing sleep; and antidepressants for pain, depression, and enhancing sleep [14]. Randomized clinical trials on anti-inflammatory medications (NSAIDs) such as ibuprofen or piroxicam for the management of myalgia, recommend, short-term use of these medications for analgesic and/or anti-inflammatory effects. For muscle pain, especially with stress and sleep disturbance, benzodiazepines, including diazepam and clonazepam, have been shown to be effective. Experience suggests that these are best used before bedtime to minimize sedation while awake. Cyclobenzaprine (Flexeril) has also been shown, in clinical trials of myalgia, to be efficacious in reducing pain and improving sleep and can be considered when a benzodiazepine is too sedating [15, 16]. These medications, with or without NSAIDs, can be considered for a 2–4-week trial with minimal habitual potential. However, long-term use has not been adequately tested.

Research on medications for fibromyalgia, especially with sleep disturbances, indicates that tricyclic antidepressants, such as amitriptyline (Elavil), have a significant impact on sleep disturbances, anxiety, and pain presentation in the patient. As such, long-term use of these medications has to be carefully evaluated and restricted for use in appropriate cases alone [17]. If the side effects with amitriptyline (Elavil) are significant, then nortriptyline (Pamelor) can be considered with fewer side effects. Typically, the dosage for either of these medications in these patients, without depression, is in the 25–75 mg range at bedtime. The use of selective serotonin reuptake inhibitors (SSRIs) has been suggested for depression and pain but may also have the common side effect of increasing muscle tension and aggravating the pain.

For chronic pain conditions that are resistant to interventions, use of opioids can be considered. Tramadol has been shown to be effective in fibromyalgia. Presently, chronic opioid use is mainly indicated for patients with chronic intractable severe pain conditions that are refractory to all other reasonable treatments because of their side effects, including constipation, sedation, potential for dose escalation, and unknown effects with long-term use.

Despite the advantages of medications for pain disorders, there exists an opportunity for problems to occur due to their misuse. The problems that can occur from the use of medications include chemical dependency, behavioral reinforcement of continuing pain, and inhibition of endogenous pain relief mechanisms, side effects, and adverse effects from the concurrent use of multiple medications.

Control of Contributing Factors

Identifying and addressing the contributing factors associated with myofascial pain is a very important step in the management of the condition with significant prognostic implication.

Behavioral Factors

There are spinal postural factors as well as oro-mandibular postural factors that play a significant role in influencing myofascial pain. Postural factors could be behavioral or biological in origin. For example, prolonged periods of sustaining forward head posture can result in foreshortening of the muscles and hyperextension of ligaments and muscles, and the resulting misalignment can predispose the head and neck region to injury. The oro-mandibular posture, wherein the mandible rests in a protrusive and/or clenched occlusal relationship with the maxilla, can result in significantly altered muscle tone at rest also predisposing the masticatory unit to myofascial injury. Behaviorally, altered spinal posture can occur with poor computer station ergonomics, phone-cradling between the head and the shoulder, and texting and operating digital media in forward head posture. Altered oro-mandibular posture could result from oral parafunctional habits such as teeth clenching bruxism, nail-biting, lip-biting, and cheek biting. Repetitive strain from activities such as gum chewing could also influence the masticatory myofascial pain.

Elevated muscle tone and muscle tension being the underlying factors that tie these behavioral factors to myofascial pain, treatment approaches aimed at addressing muscle tension such as the management of stress and anxiety with the use of counseling, relaxation techniques and biofeedback needs to be front and center in the overall management strategy. While the awareness about these behavioral factors is the first step to addressing these contributing factors, long-term success cannot be ensured with habit reversal technique alone and needs to be supplemented with a comprehensive array of treatment approaches that address the above mentioned conditions influencing the underlying muscle tension.

Summary

Myofascial pain is a chronic recurrent condition. Setting short-term and long-term goals with appropriate treatment approaches is necessary given the risk of chronicity with the condition. After establishing the complexity of the condition based on its clinical severity, an array of treatment options are available to carefully tailor to the patient's needs. A positive doctor–patient relationship with a multidisciplinary team of healthcare professionals, addressing both the clinical symptoms and the contributing factors, is important to achieve success with the treatment. Success with the treatment is accomplished when the patient becomes independent in the day-to-day management of the condition, as he or she integrates the skills gained with the various treatment approaches to his or her lifestyle.

Acknowledgement None declared.

Conflict of Interest None declared.

References

1. Okeson JP. Bell's orofacial pains. 5th ed. Chicago: Quintessence; 1995.
2. Fricton J, Kroening R, Haley D, Siegert R. Myofascial pain syndrome of the head and neck: a review of clinical characteristics of 164 patients. Oral Surg Oral Med Oral Pathol. 1985;60:615.
3. Fricton JR. Myofascial pain syndrome: characteristics and epidemiology. In: Fricton JR, Awad EA, editors. Myofascial pain and fibromyalgia. New York: Raven Press; 1990.
4. Skootsky S, Jaeger B, Oye RK. Prevalence of myofascial pain in general internal medicine practice. West J Med. 1989;151:157.
5. Fricton JR. Recent advances in temporomandibular disorders and orofacial pain. J Am Dent Assoc. 1991;122:24 [see comments].
6. Travell J, Simons DG. Myofascial pain and dysfunction: the trigger point manual. Baltimore, MA: Williams & Wilkins; 1998.
7. Simons D. Muscular pain syndromes. In: Fricton JR, Awad EA, editors. Myofascial pain and fibromyalgia. New York: Raven Press; 1990.
8. Okeson JP, editor. Orofacial pain: guidelines for assessment, diagnosis, and management. Chicago: Quintessence; 1996.
9. Lund JP, Donga R, Widmer CG, Stohler CS. The pain-adaptation model: a discussion of the relationship between chronic musculoskeletal pain and motor activity. Can J Physiol Pharmacol. 1991;69:683.
10. Dall Arancio D, Friction J. Randomized controlled study of exercises for masticatory myofascial pain. J Orofac Pain. 1993;7:117.
11. Shata R, Mehta NR, Forgione AG. Active resistance exercise for TMD related tension pain. J Dent Res 2000;79:abstr. 3541.
12. Au AR, Klineberg IJ. Isokinetic exercise management of temporomandibular joint clicking in young adults. J Prosthet Dent. 1993;70:33.
13. Magnusson T, Syren M. Therapeutic jaw exercises and interocclusal appliance therapy: a comparison between two common treatments of temporomandibular disorders. Swed Dent J. 1999;23:27.
14. Fields HL, Liebeskind JC, editors. Pharmacological approaches to the treatment of chronic pain: new concepts and critical issues. Seattle, WA: IASP Press; 1994.
15. Dionne RA. Pharmacologic treatments for temporomandibular disorders. Oral Surg Oral Med Oral Pathol Oral Radiol Endod. 1997;83:134.
16. Singer E, Dionne R. A controlled evaluation of ibuprofen and diazepam for chronic orofacial muscle pain. J Orofac Pain. 1997;11:139.
17. Wedel A, Carlsson GE. Sick-leave in patients with functional disturbances of the masticatory system. Swed Dent J. 1987;11:53.

Index

A
Acetaminophen
  dosage, 82–83
  NAPQI, 82
Adaptation, psychological, 94
Ad fibers, 29
Adjuvants. *See* Analgesics and adjuvants, age groups
Advanced sleep phase syndrome, 41
Adverse effects, local anesthesia
  localized, 75–76
  systemic, medications, 77
Ageusia, 11
AHI. *See* Apnea–hypopnea index (AHI)
Allodynia, 2
Alternative sleep scoring/staging, 40
American academy of orofacial pain guidelines, 15
American Academy of Sleep Medicine (AASM), 54
American Board of Medical Hypnosis (ABMH), 130
American Geriatrics Society (AGS) guidelines, 85
American Society of Clinical Hypnosis (ASCH), 129, 130
Anaesthesiol, E.J., 153
Analgesics and adjuvants, age groups
  chronic pain, 81
  pain formulary considerations
    pediatric/obstetrical/elderly patients, 84
    pregnant female patient, 85
  pharmacologic management, elderly
    AGS guidelines, 85
    cognitive approaches, 86
    opioids, 86
    side effects, 86

WHO analgesic ladder
  step 1: analgesics for mild pain, 82–83
  step 2: analgesics for moderate pain, 83
  step 3: severe pain, 83–84
Anesthesia conduction, 65, 72
Ankyloglossia, 11
Anosmia, 9
Anticonvulsants, 146. *See also* Paroxysmal neuralgia, pain management
Aphthous stomatitis, 103
Apne–ahypopnea index (AHI), 44
ASCH. *See* American Society of Clinical Hypnosis (ASCH)
Ashburn, M.A., 153
Asthma, 43
Autoadjusting positive airway pressure (APAP), 57

B
Bakken, E., 115
Berger, T., 36
Bilevel positive airway pressure (BiPAP), 57
Biofeedback technique, 128–129
Bradley, L.A., 95
Braid, J., 116
Bruxism, 123
Bupivacaine, 66
Burning mouth syndrome (BMS)
  causes, 104
  complications, 108
  definitions, 105
  diagnostic tests, 110
  risk factors, 107
  symptoms, 107
  tests and diagnosis, 109–110
  treatments and drugs, 111–112

C

Calcitoin gene-related peptide (CGRP), 25
Central, atypical odontalgia
    clinical features, 149
    management, 149
    "phantom tooth pain", 149
    "toothache of unknown cause", 149
Central nervous system sensitization, 10
Central relay, neuralgia
    thalamus, 3
    trigeminal spinal tract nucleus
        subnucleus caudalis, 3
        subnucleus interpolaris, 3
        subnucleus oralis, 3
Central sleep apnea (CSA) syndrome, 44–45
C fibers, 29
CGRP. *See* Calcitoin gene-related peptide (CGRP)
"Charley horse". *See* Sleep-related leg cramps
Chemonociceptors, 26
Cholecystokinin (CCK), 25
Chronic obstructive pulmonary disease (COPD), 43
Chronic pain, 81
Chronic Pain Battery, 165
Circadian rhythm sleep disorders (CRSD), 46
Classification, orofacial pain
    American academy of orofacial pain guidelines, 15
    "differential diagnosis", 15
    IASP, 15
    ICD10—G 50.0 disorders of trigeminal nerve, 15
    RDC/TMD, 15
Cluster headache
    chronic, 138
    clinical presentation and diagnosis, 138
    epidemiology, 139
    episodic, 138
    pathogenesis, 139
    signs or symptoms, 138
    treatment
        pharmacologic, 139
        prophylactic therapies, 139
        surgical intervention, 139–140
Cognitive behavioral therapy (CBT)
    benefits, 100
    characteristics
        brief and time limited, 91
        cognitive distortions, 93
        cognitive restructuring, 94–95
        educational model, 92
        emotional response, 91
        goal achievement, 92–93
        inductive method, 92
        pain management modalities, 93–94
        patient-oriented group sessions, 93
        randomized, controlled studies, 95
        Socratic method, 92
        stoic philosophy, 92
        structured and directive, 92
        therapeutic relationship, 91
        therapist and patient, 91
        training, 94, 95
    cognitive distortions, 99
    goals, 99
    pain condition, 99
    pain management
        assessment, 97
        guidelines, 97
        medical care, 98
        recurrence, 95
        risks, 98–100
        sessions, 98
        skills, 99
    stages of change and clinician's tasks, 96
    steps (typical)
        conditions and issues, 94, 96
        negative or inaccurate patient thinking, 96–97
        patient's thoughts and beliefs, 95–96
    stress and physical interactions
        headache, 90
        low back pain, 90
        neck pain (myofascial pain), 90
        pain and stress, 91
        TMD, 90
Cognitive distortions, 99
Cold sores/blisters, 104
Continuous neuropathic pain
    central, atypical odontalgia
        clinical features, 149
        management, 149
        "phantom tooth pain", 149
        "toothache of unknown cause", 149
    pathophysiology
        central sensitization, 147
        neuroplasticity, 147
        peripheral sensitization, 147
    peripheral continuous neuropathic pain
        deafferentation pain, 148–149
        neuritis pain, 148
Continuous positive airway pressure (CPAP), 57
Crain, J., 115–131
Cranial nerves, 155
CRSD. *See* Circadian rhythm sleep disorders (CRSD)

Index

D
Dabu-Bondoc, S., 1–6, 25–31
David, J., 15–21
Deafferentation pain
 clinical features, 148
 management, 149
Dental local anesthetics
 non-injectable, 66
 techniques of administration
  anterior superior alveolar nerve block, 73
  inferior alveolar nerve, 73–74
  infiltration techniques, 72
  infraorbital nerve block, 73
  maxillary nerve block (V2 block), 73
  middle superior alveolar nerve block, 72
  nasopalatine block, 73
  nerve block anesthesia, 72
  oral and maxillofacial surgery procedures, 74–75
  palatine nerve block, 73
  PDL technique (intraligamentary injection), 74
  posterior superior alveolar nerve block, 72
  trigeminal nerve, 74–75
Dental pulp, 2, 17
Dental sleep medicine and oral devices
 alternative sleep scoring/staging, 40
 clinical assessment, 54–56
 cycles and hours of sleep, 40–41
 fibromyalgia (FM), 53
 gastroesophageal reflux, 53
 headache disorders, 51–53
 idiopathic atypical odontalgia, 51
 myofacial pain, 50
 oral and maxillofacial surgery (telegnathic surgery), 61
 orofacial pain, 50
 pain and sleep, 49–50
 REM sleep, 39–40
 RFVTR, 60
 sleep apnea management/treatment, 57–60
 sleep architect, 36–39
 sleep disorders and assessment, 42–49
 sleep–wake cycle, 41–42
 subjective self-assessment, 54
 temporal arteritis (TA), 51
 temporomandibular disorders, 50
 toothache, 51
 trigeminal and glossopharyngeal neuralgia, 50
Diphenhydramine (Benadryl), 110

E
EAAs. *See* Excitatory amino acids (EAAs)
EEG. *See* Electroencephalogram (EEG)
Electroencephalogram (EEG), 37
Electroencephalography, discovery, 36
Electromyography (EMG), 37
Electrooculography (EOG), 37
EMG. *See* Electromyography (EMG)
EOG. *See* Electrooculography (EOG)
Epidemiology, 16
Episodic neuropathic pain
 neurovascular pain, 144
 paroxysmal neuralgia, 144–147
EPSPs. *See* Excitatory postsynaptic potentials (EPSPs)
Epworth Sleepiness Scale, 54
Excitatory amino acids (EAAs), 29
Excitatory postsynaptic potentials (EPSPs), 30

F
"Facial Pain Not Fulfilling Other Criteria", 5
Femiano, F., 106
Fibromyalgia (FM)
 alpha–delta sleep, 53
 criteria, 53
 widespread muscle pain presentation, 163
Finger focus technique
 children, 127
 self-hypnosis, 126
FM. *See* Fibromyalgia (FM)

G
GABA, inhibitory neurotransmitter, 4
Gag reflex
 and orofacial pain management, 124, 125
 pain reduction, 124–125
 self-hypnosis technique, 125–126
 tinnitus, 124
Gastroesophageal reflux, 53
General anesthesia (GA), 65
Giant cell arteritis. *See* Temporal arteritis (TA)
Giri, S., 143–149, 161–171
Glossopharyngeal neuralgia (GN), 18
GN. *See* Glossopharyngeal neuralgia (GN)
Gottschalk, A, 153
Gowda, A.M., 25–31
Gruenbaum, S., 1–6

H

Halaszynski, T.M., 65–78, 89–100, 103–112
Headache
  biofeedback, 128
  facial pain and ulceration, 123
Headache disorders
  chronic daily, 51–53
  cluster headache, 52
  habitual snoring, 52
  hypnic headache, 52
  ICSD-2, 52
  insomnia, 52
  migraine attacks, 52
  morning headaches, 51–53
  sleep hygiene, 52
  sleep-related headaches, 52–53
  temporal or tension-type headaches, 52
Herpetiform ulcers, 104, 106
Hickey, A.H., 81–86
Huang, Y., 1–6
Hydrodynamic mechanism, 26
Hyperalgesia, 2
Hypersomnias
  narcolepsy with cataplexy, 45
  narcolepsy without cataplexy, 46
Hypnosis
  bruxism, 123
  chemotherapy treatments, 115, 116
  dental practice, 122
  emotional roadblocks, treatment, 121
  fears/phobias, 119
  gag reflex, 123–126
  "induction", 118
  medical/dental practice, 117–118
  misconceptions, 117
  relaxation, 118–119
  state of mind, 120–121
  subconscious and conscious, 116
  treatment fear, 122–123

I

IASP. *See* International Association for the Study of Pain (IASP)
ICD10—G 50.0 disorders of trigeminal nerve, 15
Idiopathic atypical odontalgia, 51
Imagery biofeedback, 119–120
Insomnias
  definition, 36, 43
  excessive daytime sleepness (EDS), 43
  PSG sleep study, 43
International Association for the Study of Pain (IASP), 15, 95, 143

International Classification of Sleep Disorders (ICSD), 42
International Headache Society (IHS), 133
Intravenous (IV) sedation, 65
Iyengar, S., 153

J

Jensen, M., 126

K

Kai, A., 25–31
Kaspo, G.A., 35–62, 133–140
Kaye, A.D., 151–160

L

Laser-assisted UPPP (LAUP), 60
Laughlin, I., 81–86
Lichen planus, 106
Lidocaine, 66
Local anesthesia
  cardiovascular system, 78
  central nervous system, 77–78
  classification, 66, 67
  definition, 66
  dental local anesthetics (*see also* Dental local anesthetics)
    non-injectable, 66
    techniques of administration, 72–75
  hypersensitivity/allergy, 77
  injectable, 66
  ion trapping, 69
  localized adverse effects, 75–76
  mechanism of action, 66–69
  "membrane-stabilizing" drugs, 68
  needle placement techniques, risks, 76
  nerve conduction, 68, 69
  para-aminobenzoic acid (PABA), 76
  pharmacokinetics, 67
  properties, 68, 69
  recovery and causes, 76–77
  state-dependent blockade, 68
  structure, 66, 67
  systemic adverse effects from medications, 77
  techniques of administration
    field block, 71
    infiltration anesthesia, 71
    injections/nerve block techniques, 69, 70
    peripheral nerve block, 71
    plexus anesthesia, 71
    surface anesthesia, 70

topical anesthetics, 66
treatment of overdose: "lipid rescue", 78
undesired effects, 75
Low back pain, 90

M
Maintenance of wakefulness test (MWT), 56–57
Mancini, P., 1–6
Masticatory myofascial pain
  clinical presentation, 162–163
  etiologic factors
    direct or indirect macro-trauma, 163
    occupational and repetitive strain injury, 164
    oral parafunctional habits, 164
  masticatory myalgia, 161
  pain
    active trigger point, 162
    comorbid conditions and contributing factors, 163
    fibromyalgia, 163
    latent trigger point, 162
    limited range of motion, 162
    muscle tenderness, 162
    other symptoms, 162–163
    tender points, 163
    trigger points, 162
    "zone of reference", 162
  pathophysiology and mechanisms
    central biasing mechanism, 164
    central hypotheses, 164
    Chronic Pain Battery, 165
    diagnostic tests, 165
    neurophysiological hypothesis, 164
    repetitive strain hypotheses, 164
    TMJ Scale, 165
  treatment (see Masticatory pain, treatment)
  trigger points, 161
Masticatory pain, treatment
  control of contributing factors
    altered oro-mandibular posture, 171
    behavioral factors, 171
  orthopedic intraoral splints
    anterior repositioning splints, 167
    habit reversal, 168
    mandibular splints, 167
  palliative self-care program for acute episodes, 167
  pharmacotherapy
    analgesics, 170
    medications for fibromyalgia, 170
    selective serotonin reuptake inhibitors (SSRIs), 170
    tramadol, 170
  physical therapy exercises
    corrective postural guidance, 168
    muscle stretching, 168
    postural awareness and training, 168
  physical therapy modalities, 169–170
  self-care, 166–167
  simple to complex
    CBT, 165
    TENS, 165
    treatment goals, 166
  trigger point dry needling, 169
  trigger point injections, 169
Maxillomandibular advancement surgery (MMA), 61
Mechano-nociceptors, 26
Methadone, 84
MFP. See Myofacial pain (MFP)
Migraine headaches
  chronic, 136
  epidemiology, 136–137
  with or without aura, 136
  pain characteristics, 136
  pathogenesis, 137
  status migrainosus, 136
  treatment
    acute migraine, 137
    nonpharmacologic, 137
    pharmacologic, 137
    preventive treatments, 137–138
MMA. See Maxillomandibular advancement surgery (MMA)
Moskowitz, M.A., 137
Mouth rehabilitation, 10
Mouthwashes, 109
MSLT. See Multiple sleep latency test (MSLT)
Multimodal polypharmacy, 82
Multiple sleep latency test (MSLT), 56
Muscle stretching exercises, masticatory pain, 168
Myofacial pain (MFP), 50

N
N-acetyl-p-benzoquinone imine (NAPQI), 82
Neck pain (myofascial pain), 90
Nerve block techniques. See Dental local anesthetics
Neuralgia(s)
  GN, 18
  paroxysmal (see Paroxysmal neuralgia, pain management)
  PHN, 18, 48
  sphenopalatine neuralgia, 18
  TN, 18

Neuritis pain
  clinical features, 148
  management
    post-herpetic neuralgia, 148
    source of infection, 148
Neurobiology of orofacial pain
  biochemical influences
    c-Fos, 4
    GABA, 4
    GABA(A) receptors, 4
    GABA(B) receptors, 4
    NADPH, 4
    neurons, 4
    nitric oxide (NO), 4
  central relay, 3
  modulation, 2
  neuropathic orofacial pain
    atypical facial pain, 5
    insidious pain, 5
    nerve damage, 5
    neuronal injury, 5
    trigeminal, 5
    vascular pain, 5
  primary afferent nociceptor, 2
  TMJ disorders, 6
Neurons, 4
Neuropathic pain, definition, 143
Neurotransmitter agents
NMDA. See N-Methyl-D-Aspartate (NMDA) receptor
N-Methyl-D-Aspartate (NMDA) receptor, 30
Nociceptive chemical mediators, oral inflammation
  conduction
    Ad fibers, first pain, 29
    C fibers, second pain, 29
    EAAs, 29
  pathophysiology of orofacial pain, 26–27
  transduction
    acute tissue injury, 28
    primary and secondary noxious sensitizers, 27–28
    receptor–G-protein complex, 28
    substance P, 28
  transmission
    definition, 29
    EPSPs, 30
    excitatory amino acids, 29–30
    frequency stimulation, 29
    NMDA receptor, 30
    Rexed's laminae II, 29
Nociceptors
  chemonociceptors, 26
  mechano-nociceptors, 26
  substance P, 2, 26
  thermo-nociceptors, 26
Non-Hodgkin's lymphoma, 115
Non-REM (NREM)
  N1, light sleep, 36, 37
  N2, consolidated sleep, 37–38
  N3, deep or slow-wave sleep, 37, 38
  states of sleep, 36–38
Nonsteroidal anti-inflammatory drugs (NSAIDs), 83
Non-tooth-related orofacial pain
  cardiac toothache, 20
  headache, 20
  idiopathic, 19
  neuralgias, 18
  neuropathic, 18
  painful oral mucosal lesions, 19
  psychosomatic diseases, 19
  salivary gland diseases, 20
  sinonasal diseases, 19–20
  TMD, 17–18
Novocain. See Local anesthesia
NREM. See Non-REM (NREM)
NSAIDs. See Nonsteroidal anti-inflammatory drugs (NSAIDs)

O

Obstructive sleep apnea (OSA)
  complete (apnea), 45
  partial (hypopnea), 45
  surgical treatment, 60
  syndrome, 44, 45
Olness, K., 129
μ-Opioid agonists, 84
Opioids, 83–84
Oral and maxillofacial surgery (telegnathic surgery), 61
Oral appliance (OA) therapy, 41, 59
Oral health impact profile (OHIP), 12
Oral health-related quality of life (OHRQoL)
  components, 9
  dental education, 12
  facial disorders/pain
    ageusia, 11
    ankyloglossia, 11
    cleft lip and palate, 11
    jaw fractures, 10
    migraine, 11
    radiotherapy and surgery, oral/nasal cancer, 11
    stroke, 10
    TMD, 10
  general health, 10

indices, 12
qualitative research, 12
Oral inflammation. *See* Nociceptive chemical mediators, oral inflammation
Oral ulcers
  alpha-lipoic acid, 105
  aphthae, 103
  aphthous ulcers, major/minor, 104, 106
  cold sores/blisters, 104
  complications, 108
  definitions, 103
  herpetiform ulcers, 104, 106
  lower lip, 104
  risk factors, 107
  symptoms, 106
  systemic and iatrogenic causes, 104
  tests and diagnosis, 108–109
  treatments and drugs, 110–111
  trench mouth (Vincent's stomatitis), 104
Orofacial neuropathic pain, management
  classification, 143–144
  continuous neuropathic pain, 147–148
  episodic neuropathic pain, 144–147
Orofacial pain management
  ABMH, 130
  ASCH, 129
  biofeedback technique, 128–129
  cyberphysiology, 115
  hypnosis (*see* Hypnosis)
  self-hypnosis induction techniques, 126–128
Orthognathic surgery, 60
OSA. *See* Obstructive sleep apnea (OSA)

P

Pain and sleep, 49–50
Para-aminobenzoic acid (PABA), 76
Parasomnias, 36, 46–47
Paroxysmal hemicrania, 140
Paroxysmal neuralgia, pain management
  clinical features
    trigeminal neuralgia, 145
    "trigger zone", 145
  neurosurgical treatment strategies
    peripheral radiofrequency thermolysis, 146
    rhizotomy, 147
  paroxysmal pain, 145
  pathophysiology, 145
  pharmacological treatment strategies
    carbamazepine, anticonvulsant, 146
    gabapentin, 146
    "trigger zone", 146

Pathophysiology, orofacial pain
  chemo-nociceptors, 26
  hydrodynamic mechanism, 26
  mechano-nociceptors, 26
  primary peripheral afferents, 26
  thermo-nociceptors, 26
  trigeminal nerve
    subnucleus caudalis, 26
    subnucleus oralis and interpolaris, 26–27
Periodic limb movement disorder (PLMD), 47–48
Periodic limb movement sleep (PLMS), 47–48
Peripheral continuous neuropathic pain
  deafferentation pain, 148–149
  neuritis pain, 148
"Phantom tooth pain", 149
PLMD. *See* Periodic limb movement disorder (PLMD)
Polysomnography (PSG), 54–55
Positive airway pressure (PAP) therapy
  autoadjusting positive airway pressure (APAP), 57
  bilevel positive airway pressure (BiPAP), 57
  continuous positive airway pressure (CPAP), 57
Postherpetic neuralgia (PHN), 18
Primary afferent nociceptor
  Aβ fibers, 2
  Aδ fibers, 2
  C fibers, 2
  chemo-nociceptors, 2
  mechanonociceptors, 2
  thermo-nociceptors, 2
Primary headache, 133
Procaine, 66
Prostaglandin (PGE), 25
PSG. *See* Polysomnography (PSG)
Public health, population, 9, 12

Q

Quality of life, 9

R

Radiofrequency volumetric tissue reduction (RFVTR), 60
Rapid eye movement (REM)
  dream sleep, 39
  paradoxical sleep, Europe, 42
  stage R, 39
  states of sleep, 36
  tonic and phasic, 40

RDC/TMD. *See* Research diagnostic criteria for temporomandibular diseases (RDC/TMD)
RDI. *See* Respiratory disturbance index (RDI)
Receptors, 25, 28–29
Recurrent aphthous stomatitis, 103
Relaxation, breathing, 118–119, 126
REM. *See* Rapid eye movement (REM)
Research diagnostic criteria for temporomandibular diseases (RDC/TMD), 15
Respiratory disturbance index (RDI), 44
Restless legs syndrome (RLS), 47
RFVTR. *See* Radiofrequency volumetric tissue reduction (RFVTR)
Rhizotomy, 147. *See also* Paroxysmal neuralgia, pain management
RLS. *See* Restless legs syndrome (RLS)

S
Selective serotonin reuptake inhibitors (SSRIs), 170
Self-hypnosis induction techniques
  finger focus technique, 126–127
  intentional thinking, 127–128
  medical/dental practice, 126
  relaxation breathing, 126
Setty, S., 15–21
Shulman, J., 129
Sleep apnea, management/treatment
  behavioral management, 57
  dental appliances
    FDA document, 59
    mandibular advancement splints, 59
    OA therapy, 59
    TMJ dysfunction, 59–60
    TRD and MAD, 59
    treatment of OSA, 58–59
  medical treatment
    CPAP, 58
    PAP therapy, 57–58
  surgical treatment, OSA, 60
  UPPP and LAUP, 60
Sleep bruxism, 42, 48–49, 52
Sleep, cycles and hours
  advanced sleep phase syndrome, 41
  normal sleep, 40
  slow-wave sleep, 40
  SRBD, 41
Sleep disorders and assessment
  breathing disorders
    central sleep apnea syndrome, 44–45
    hypersomnias, 45
    OSA syndromes, 44, 45
    snoring, 43–44
  circadian rhythm sleep disorders, 46
  hypersomnias
    narcolepsy with cataplexy, 45
    narcolepsy without cataplexy, 46
  insomnias, 36, 43
  movement disorders
    medical conditions, 49
    PLMD, 47–48
    RLS, 47
    sleep-related leg cramps, 48
    SRB, 48–49
  parasomnias, 36, 46–47
Sleep-related bruxism (SRB), 48–49
Sleep-related leg cramps, 48
Sleep–wake cycle
  circadian rhythm
    24-h process C, 41
    temperature recordings, 41
  schedule disorders, 36
  ultradian rhythm
    apnea and hypopnea, 42
    atonia, 42
    24-h process C, 41–42
    sleep bruxism, 42
    sleep disorders, 42
    sleep stages 1 and 2, light sleep, 42
    stages 3 and 4, deep sleep, 42
Smith, D., 153
Snoring, 43–44
Soft tissue oral facial pain
  examination, 109
  history, 109
Somnoplasty, 60
Spagnoli, D.B., 151–160
Sphenopalatine neuralgia, 18
SRB. *See* Sleep-related bruxism (SRB)
SSRIs. *See* Selective serotonin reuptake inhibitors (SSRIs)
Substance P (sP), 25–26
Syrjala, K.L., 95

T
Temporal arteritis (TA), 51
Temporomandibular disorders/ dysfunction (TMD), 10, 50
Temporomandibular joint (TMJ) disorders
  genetic risk factors, 6
  symptoms, 6
  TMD, 6
"Tender points", 163

TENS. *See* Transcutaneous electrical nerve stimulations (TENS)
Tension-type headache (TTH)
  categories
    frequent headaches, 133
    infrequent headaches, 133
    new daily persistent headache, 133
  chronic TTH (CTTH), 134
  clinical presentation and diagnosis, 133–134
  epidemiology, 134
  episodic, 135
  muscle contraction or tension headache, 134
  pathogenesis, 134–135
  treatment
    over-the-counter analgesics, 135
    pharmacotherapy, 135
    simple analgesics, 135
Tetracaine, 66
Thermo-nociceptors, 26
Thorp, S., 25–31
Tinnitus, 124
TMJ Scale, 165
Tongue-retaining device (TRD), 59
Toothache, 51
"Toothache of unknown cause", 149
Tooth-related orofacial pain
  acute periapical abscess, 17
  cracked or fractured tooth, 17
  dental decay, 17
Transcutaneous electrical nerve stimulations (TENS), 165
Trench mouth (Vincent's stomatitis), 104
Trigeminal and glossopharyngeal neuralgia, 50
Trigeminal autonomic cephalalgia, 133
Trigeminal neuralgia (TN), 18
Trigger point, masticatory myofascial pain
  active, 162
  dry needling, 169
  latent, 162
  point injections, 169
Turner, J.A., 95

U
Upper airway resistance syndrome (UARS), 57
Uvulopalatopharyngoplasty (UPPP), 60

V
Vadivelu, A., 1–6, 9–13, 25–31
Vadivelu, N., 1–6, 25–31
Vasoconstriction, 65, 66

W
WHO analgesic ladder. *See also* Analgesics and adjuvants, age groups
  step 1: analgesics for mild pain
    acetaminophen
    NSAIDs, 83
  step 2: analgesics for moderate pain, 83
  step 3: severe pain
    methadone, 84
    μ-Opioid agonists, 84
    opioids, 83–84
Woolf, C.J., 30

Y
Yapko, M.D., 118
Yawning, 10, 164

Z
"Zone of reference", 162